T0144594

# NEW APPROACHES IN SOCIOLOGY
## STUDIES IN SOCIAL INEQUALITY, SOCIAL CHANGE, AND SOCIAL JUSTICE

*Edited By*
## Nancy Naples
University of Connecticut

# A ROUTLEDGE SERIES

# New Approaches in Sociology

Studies in Social Inequality, Social Change, and Social Justice

Nancy Naples, *General Editor*

# TALKING BACK TO PSYCHIATRY
## The Psychiatric
## Consumer/Survivor/Ex-Patient Movement

Linda J. Morrison

Routledge
New York & London

Published in 2005 by
Routledge
Taylor & Francis Group
270 Madison Ave,
New York NY 10016

Published in Great Britain by
Routledge
Taylor & Francis Group
2 Park Square,
Milton Park, Abingdon,
Oxon, OX14 4RN

© 2005 by Taylor & Francis Group, LLC
Routledge is an imprint of Taylor & Francis Group.

Transferred to Digital Printing 2009

International Standard Book Number-10: 0-415-97305-8 (Hardcover)
International Standard Book Number-13: 978-0-415-97305-2 (Hardcover)
Library of Congress Card Number 2004027819

---

### Library of Congress Cataloging-In-Publication Data

---

Morrison, Linda Joy.
    Talking back to psychiatry : the psychiatric consumer/survivor/ex-patient movement / Linda Joy Morrison.
        p. cm. -- (New approaches in sociology)
    Includes bibliographical references and index.
    ISBN: 0-415-97305-8 (hardback)
    1. Antipsychiatry—Social aspects—United States. 2. Ex-mental patients—Civil rights—United States. 3. Mentally ill—Civil rights—United States. 4. Mental illness—Social aspects—United States. 5. Mentally ill—Social conditions—United States. 6. Ex-mental patients—Social conditions—United States. I. Title. II. Series.

RC437.5.M66 2005
362.196'89--dc22                                         2004027819

---

ISBN10: 0-415-97305-8 (hbk)
ISBN10: 0-415-80489-2 (pbk)

ISBN13: 978-0-415-97305-2 (hbk)
ISBN13: 978-0-415-80489-9 (pbk)

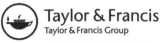

**Taylor & Francis**
Taylor & Francis Group

LONDON AND NEW YORK
Taylor & Francis Group
is the Academic Division of T&F Informa plc.

**Visit the Taylor & Francis Web site at
http://www.taylorandfrancis.com**

**and the Routledge Web site at
http://www.routledge-ny.com**

# Contents

# Acknowledgments

I wish to thank all the people who made this project possible and encouraged me to do the work. Many thanks to my friends in the movement who have shared their lives and passions in order to help me understand. I owe it all to you. Thanks to my department colleagues and Kathleen Blee for their encouragement and support. Thanks especially to the people who inspired me but are no longer here to share the joy: Nancy Abel, Jim Alles, Jack Barry, Diana Forsythe, Ron Gibson, Joyce King, Fred Koloc, and Steve Sapolsky. I hope they are smiling somewhere in peace. Thanks to the dear friends who helped me through it: Suzanne, Paul and Rachel, Penny and Phil, Kellee and Saul, Jean-Luc, Ken and Brad, dear patient Fred who was so supportive, and Jeff who proved it was possible. Many thanks to all the activists, who know the work is not over yet. To my daughter Anna, whose mom has been a student nearly all her 25 years, thanks for letting me finish first. And above all I thank my parents, Alan and Joy, who believed in me.

# Introduction

## THE CONSUMER/SURVIVOR/EX-PATIENT MOVEMENT

This research was designed to learn about the experience and motivations of activists in the psychiatric consumer/survivor/ex-patient (c/s/x) movement. Most members of the c/s/x movement are people who have been diagnosed as mentally ill and are engaged in different forms of "talking back" to psychiatry and the mental health system. Other activists include dissident mental health professionals, lawyers, advocates, and family members: allies who have may not have been diagnosed and treated (psychiatrized) but support the movement's efforts to challenge the current practices of psychiatry and the existing system of mental health treatment. The term "psychiatry" is used within the movement to refer to the standard biomedical and psychopharmacological models of practice that shape the mental health system and are generally used by psychiatrists and ancillary mental health practitioners.

Members of the c/s/x movement are not satisfied to settle into the ordinary sick role (Parsons 1951) or accept the deviant "mental patient" identity (Scheff 1999) assigned to them by their doctors and society. Instead, they adopt an alternative point of view. They work to take power in relation to their providers, and attempt to shape treatment to respond to their own needs or reject it altogether. They also work to empower others in similar ways, both through individual advocacy and by organized efforts to change the system at local and national levels. For these activists, the constraints of the mental health system and standard treatment practice are the problems that require solution, rather than the problems posed by their "mental illness" and their "sick" selves. Instead of being passive objects of treatment, policy and social control, they take an activist stance toward increased alternatives, informed choice, and human rights protection for people who find themselves within the power domain of psychiatric care.

This book explores the ways in which movement activists "talk back" in response to the power, knowledge and expectations of psychiatry, and how this resistant response differs from the internalization of mental patient identity described by Thomas Scheff in *Becoming Mentally Ill* (1999). I focused on their experiences of being "mental patients" and their relationship to psychiatric practice, with particular focus on problems of fit between their own experience of what they need and what they find helpful in solving their problems, as well as the constraints and expectations imposed on them by psychiatry's "expert knowledge" definitions of who they are and what they need. I then explore how they respond to these disparities through enacting resistant identities and engaging in advocacy to address the imbalance of power through direct and indirect means. By participating in activities of the larger social movement at regional and national levels, activists benefit from emotional support and technical assistance that strengthen their activism on the local level. An awareness of collective goals and a sense of solidarity with the ongoing mission of change and empowerment build their identity as part of a larger historical movement of resistance and change.

People who work to advocate for others in the mental health system talk about resisting psychiatry on the personal level as well. They challenge the authority of their doctors to define them as "a diagnosis" and to determine their needs according to "best practices" of treatment for these diagnostic labels. Instead of being passive patients, they place themselves in the more active, resistant, and self-defined roles of "consumers," "survivors," or "ex-patients" of psychiatry.

This book also explores the meaning of these roles to movement participants, and how they reflect various ways to "talk back" and resist the power of psychiatry to define and constrain their lives. As psychiatric consumers, they demand information and choice in the treatment relationship. As survivors, they refer to surviving psychiatric treatment and moving beyond it. As ex-patients, they refuse the patient role. All of these terms reflect positions of increased power in relation to psychiatry. Throughout its history the c/s/x movement has promoted resistance, solidarity and collective strength among its members to challenge psychiatry's dominance in various ways in different social contexts. The goal of my work is to contribute to a deeper understanding of the movement and its members, meanings and processes.

The consumer/survivor/ex-patient (c/s/x) movement's cumbersome multi-part name has personified and guided much of my research. For reasons to be addressed, the inclusive "c/s/x" structure must be fully acknowledged to understand and describe the complex movement it denotes. Its persistent multiplicity has been both burdensome and revelatory for my research, providing ongoing clues about how to untangle the various points of view, identities, disputes, and tactical repertoires that underlie this multi-faceted social movement. By choosing to use this name (c/s/x) for themselves (some have recently added an "r" for recovery to the mix), I believe the c/s/x activists are emphasizing their own diversity and at the same time expressing the underlying unity of their movement.

Certainly, the complex identities and narratives at play in this movement provide insights into the experiences of people who are labeled with psychiatric diagnoses and live with the challenges of negotiating the mental health system and community life. Important issues of power and authority, of voice and personal agency, of choice and self-determination are revealed by the layers of interaction and the histories of movement participants. Beyond this, the social movement helps to illuminate the fault lines of psychiatric practice: how changing structures of power, competing interests, and shifting authority shape and define its relations to the "objects" of treatment without which it could not exist. Meanwhile, the movement stories give energy and purpose to an ongoing struggle which has continued for more than thirty years with no end in sight.

The people in the social category I have studied are not well-known to many in our society. Those who claim most knowledge of their lives and their troubles have been workers in the mental health system and family members, who tend to see and define the problems from their own points of view. So-called "mental patients" are generally feared and misunderstood by the lay public and even by many professionals. In fact it is the widespread categorization of people by psychiatric diagnosis or stereotype, and the resulting forms of treatment and dehumanization, which are the main targets for change by activists in this social movement. "Mental patients" who resist treatment and insist on speaking for themselves against mental health practices are particularly feared and misunderstood. As a collective movement, c/s/x activists have been effective in producing some changes in the mental health system while having less effect on psychiatric practice itself.

Most of the members of this movement have been diagnosed with what are called "serious and persistent mental illnesses (SPMI)." This characterization includes such psychiatric diagnoses as schizophrenia, schizoaffective (combination of thought and mood) disorder, manic-depressive or bipolar disorder, major depression, severe anxiety disorders, or some combination thereof. They have received a wide range of treatments including psychotropic drugs, hospitalizations, electroshock, seclusion and restraint, involuntary confinement and other assorted therapeutic interventions. The activists I have met in my research are speaking up about their experiences in ways and in settings that do not attract much public or media attention. Those who are aware of the issues tend to dismiss or discredit the point of view of people labeled mentally ill, although some policymakers and researchers have been more responsive to including the "consumer/survivor" point of view, in greater or lesser amounts depending on historical context as will be discussed.

In simple terms, these activists are challenging the point of view of those who diagnose and treat them. They challenge, in fact, the very use of the words in the previous paragraph including "diagnosis" (preferring "label"), "mental illness" (inserting "so-called"), and even "treatment" (inserting "so-called," using quotation marks, substituting "intervention" or "psychiatric assault"). The use of words in this movement is highly contentious, as the power to name and define the experience of the self is at stake.

The psychiatric narrative is a dominant ideology in our society; its words are not easy to challenge, especially by those it is authorized to label and define. To question this authority by providing another standpoint is a charged and political act: to demand recognition of subordinate voices, the views of the people in the movement, of those who are silenced as objects of treatment, as people who are mad. This challenge has been an ongoing process throughout the history of the c/s/x movement, and comments about the power of words will be made throughout the text.

The competing narratives of professionals, the public, and the people who are talking back in their own words about their own experience have proved a challenging and fascinating area for research. The original questions arose when my encounters with psychiatric patients and ex-patients led me to question the adequacy and relevance of Talcott Parsons' (1951) "sick role" and Scheff's (1999) "secondary deviance" in representing the relationship of these "mental patients" with psychiatry. To account for the origins of these questions, I will first explain how I came to do this research. The first chapter provides a review of the literature that has served as the intellectual background for this research project.

As a psychiatric social worker in the 1980s, I worked in a partial hospital program with people who were labeled with the serious mental illnesses listed above. At that time their psychiatric labels were referred to as "chronic" mental illnesses, and those labeled were referred to as "chronics." When the people who were called "chronics" began to talk back and complain about this derogatory usage, the term was later changed by mental health experts to "serious and persistent mental illness" in an apparent effort to be more respectful, and perhaps more scientific. Unfortunately, as a result of this change these same people are simply called "SPMI's" (as in, "Should SPMI's have children?"). The language wars (campaigns calling for "People First" language, claims that "I am a person, not a diagnosis") continue to proliferate and reveal the tensions of power dynamics, disrespect and definition.

The people attending the day treatment program where I was employed had "mental patient" identities that were firmly established after long years of socialization in the mental health system (Goffman 1961). The staff provided group and individual therapy, arts and activity groups, and skills-based groups such as assertiveness training and relaxation training. Such behaviors as medication compliance, dependency on professionals, lack of initiative, distrust of the self, and distrust of fellow "mental patients" were consistently shaped and rewarded by the staff in this traditional treatment setting.

However, other submerged or previous "pre-mentally-ill" identities were also available, even in this traditional setting. Though labeled and categorized by their diagnoses, the individual clients retained a history of unique abilities developed in earlier parts of their lives. These aspects emerged unexpectedly in activities like softball, cooking, movement, arts and music, or relaxation groups. Everyone had a history of strengths and interests they had developed before their many years of hospitalization and treatment.

For example, at softball group on Friday afternoons, a withdrawn "paranoid schizophrenic" who hadn't held a glove in years became the star fielder, outshining staff and clients alike and waving to invisible cheering crowds. A woman with a long history in the state hospital used an old family recipe to direct our lunch preparations, though her medication side effects made it impossible for her to use a knife. Frustrated artists, poets and card sharks gave us glimpses of times past.

Everyone had retained some aspects of their previous selves, even as they followed the pathways of their mental patient careers (Goffman 1961:128). These could be ignored or stifled by staff to maintain a compliant and controlled setting, or, in the right environment, they could be encouraged and celebrated. Opportunities to go beyond the limited role expectations of compliant "mental patient" gave people a chance to do more than smoke, drink coffee, and wait for the next activity group.

For me, having recently learned from "the experts" about the limited expectations of working with "low-functioning" persons, it was a source of wonder and constant revelation. There were strengths, talents, stories, and jokes, stubborn opinions, insights, and often "the clients" knew things we didn't. We had a choice about how to respond to them, and the choices made a difference. Giving up expert "control" of the situation encouraged pre-patient identities to emerge and be recognized.

With a focus on peer support and respect for persons, aided by the timely nervous breakdown of our immediate supervisor, my colleagues and I transformed our program by subverting the usual mental health system authority patterns. We invited the clients to become more active decision-makers in the program, encouraging them to choose their group activities (rather than assigned by staff), to develop peer-to-peer relationships (rather than cultivate peer distrust and encourage only vertical client-staff relations), to try out leadership roles (rather than depending on staff to give direction), to accept more responsibility in directing their own lives and helping each other.

These were effective ways to encourage underlying strengths and non-sickness-based identities. A creative and lively new peer support program was the result of our early efforts to promote this philosophy in our day-treatment setting. The former "stigma management" group became the "Don't Call Me Crazy" group, which then evolved into a client-run self-help group that fired its staff leader and held meetings off-site. Unfortunately, these creative programmatic efforts were in turn subverted by a corrective structural adjustment by the mental health bureaucracy, and the renegade program was returned to its prior state of sickness-based equilibrium after one year.

Five years later, as a graduate student in anthropology, I did participant-observation research at a peer-support-based drop-in center for mental health clients (a direct descendant of a group that started in our day treatment center). In that setting I observed a strong culture of peer support as well as a range of mixed responses to the psychiatric ideology and practice on which mental health treatment is based. Using techniques of pile-sort and cluster analysis, I found that that the value of friendship and the geographically-based community of peers (as well as music, exercise and sex) were rated much higher by participants than medication, therapy, or professional support as important sources of continued mental health and well-being.

Although the center was not a peer-run program, the client-members felt strongly that the center was their space and they had freedom with which to use it. Agency policy required that all members be seen at other sites by a psychiatrist for medication, and work with a therapist or case manager as well. Professional staff members were always on duty at the drop-in site. But the significance of these professional relationships paled beside the work groups, card games, holiday dinners, softball league trophies, and support from peers on an ongoing basis. The drop-in center was a focal point for developing "ordinary" and "non-psychiatrized" identities based on valued peer-to-peer relationships.

Moving into the intellectual framework of medical sociology, I began to think about how competing relations of power and knowledge define the experience of illness and competency, and the interplay of these competing sets of expertise in negotiating needs and treatment. The conventional scholarly wisdom in the field was represented first by Parsons' (1951) functionalist approach to the sick role, with its subsequent elaborations; and second by Scheff's (1999) delineation of labeling theory, residual deviance and internalized deviant identity, with a provocative extension into tertiary deviance by Renée Anspach (1979). Chapter one presents a discussion of these and related issues and how they shaped my research.

Chapter One
# From Sick Role to Social Movement: Theoretical Explorations

## THE SICK ROLE

Becoming "mentally ill" in a sociological sense involves the assignment of a particular social role, the "sick role" or patient role (Parsons 1951; Gerhardt 1989). As with any illness, physical or mental, the sick role includes rights and responsibilities for the person so placed: the right to be excused from normal role obligations, the right to be excused from blame for the incapacitation or illness, the obligation to seek appropriate expert assistance for the problem, and the obligation to follow through with that expert's advice. The assumption in Parsons' original explication of the sick role as elaborated by Uta Gerhardt (1989) was that proper assumption and execution of these role responsibilities would result in a return to appropriate role functioning, thus restoring social order, sparing the social system of a dysfunctional member and a threat to its stability and equilibrium. "What matters is the *social order*. Illness becomes a disturbing factor dysfunctional for the upkeep of order in society . . . the social order works on the basis of powerful homeostatic mechanisms, and medical practice is meant to constitute one, if not 'the' most important one" (1989:64).

In return, the expert caretaker has a set of reciprocal rights and responsibilities regarding the person who comes for help in the sick role process. The "doctor role" includes the right to intrude on the individual's bodily space, and the right to expect exclusive cooperation or compliance/adherence with the expert and the treatment plan. The doctor's responsibilities require putting the sick person's interests in the forefront of consideration, and using professional expertise to the greatest extent possible in the effort to cure the sick person.

The doctor is thus a "producer of care," in response to the patient's "willingness to be treated" (Gerhardt 1989:31). There is an essential inequality, an asymmetry, in the treatment situation due to the doctor's expertise and the patient's lack of it. Yet as Gerhardt points out (1989:32), it is the seeking of help by the consumer that makes the transaction possible. Thus the views of reciprocity shift according to the perceived imbalance of expertise, the desire for treatment, and the perception of treatment as social control.

The state of illness, whether physical or mental, can be seen as a form of deviance: a failure to meet normative role expectations. The moral underpinnings of this assumption are implied by Parsons' second "right" of the sick role, which is the important right not to be blamed for the illness state. This involves a moral claim that one has not brought the condition on oneself, whether by engaging in irresponsible or self-destructive behaviors such as substance abuse, reclusive self-absorption, or laziness; or, alternatively, by an overly-zealous application of socially appropriate behaviors such as overwork, over-dedication to caring for family members, or excessive spirituality. Attributions of deviance can result from an excess of positive as well as negative behaviors, either of which may be viewed as non-normative by the mainstream members of the reference group (Erikson 1966; Ben-Yehuda 1985).

For Parsons, removal of sick persons from the everyday social world is considered advantageous in a number of ways. First, it emphasizes and embodies reduced social expectations by moving the person out of the "normal" environment with its reminders of duties undone. Second, it allows for an environment of focused activities for improvement and cure. Third, removal of sick persons in their deviant state serves to prevent other members of society from observing the seductive "secondary gain" of reduced responsibilities and supportive care that are enjoyed by the persons entering the sick role. If this removal were not accomplished, the attractions of the sick role might be too hard for others to resist, causing social functioning to be further eroded. Instead, sick people are welcomed back on re-entry into everyday life when they have been cured, receiving congratulations for a successful return from a deviant state to a normal one.

In role theory, then, the temporary release from social obligations due to illness is contingent on two factors: the incapacity is involuntary, and resolution will be sought by seeking and complying with appropriate medical advice. The deviance of illness is considered undesirable and temporary, a responsible sick person is rewarded with a successful treatment, and a return to normal functioning for the individual and society is the goal.

## SICK ROLE: THE CHRONIC VARIANT

The "sick role" concept is vulnerable to critique because it does not include the realities of chronic illness. Parsons' original explication was based on a state of "acute" illness, in which a person's desire and efforts to return to health and normal social functioning would likely be successful. It failed to account for the deviance and dependency experienced by patients whose illness states were "chronic." For a person with a chronic illness, whose best help-seeking and compliant behaviors may fail to result in a return to health and normal functioning, the temporary deviant status is not resolved. Lack of resolution of the illness state necessitates a different sort of response from social actors and institutions.

In addition, chronic illnesses like diabetes, heart disease, cancer, and HIV/AIDS often lead to longer-term role changes. New social identities beyond the sick role may be required for a person who is not getting well in spite of efforts to meet the role obligations of a "good patient." These social identity negotiations include finding ways for people to remain members of society without being "put away" during an illness or disability that often will be life-long, with patterns of remission and recurrence. Kathy Charmaz (1991) has described the evolving identity issues encountered by those who do not get well, including questions of guilt, ongoing deviance, incorporating the fluctuating loss of functioning, and inability to maintain relationships.

Physicians also become frustrated and may withdraw support when their efforts at intervention fail to resolve the problem. Charles Lidz, Alan Meisel and Mark Munetz (1985) have explored ways in which new, more collaborative relationships may emerge between medical staff and patients with chronic illness. As the illness continues over time, patients develop increasing knowledge and awareness of both the illness itself and its management in their particular case. Meanwhile, as physician involvement decreases over time, opportunities for patient autonomy and self-direction of care increase. Mutual respect for differential expertise may change the balance of power, knowledge and practice in the relationship: the physician's role changes from director of care to supportive assistant, providing the technical resources needed for treating the patient's condition. Meanwhile, the patient's power and authority are enhanced in the newly-defined relationship.

## IMPLICATIONS FOR PSYCHIATRIC TREATMENT

The shifting authority, patient empowerment and validation of experiential knowledge recognized in chronic care might logically extend to psychiatric treatment, which tends to become a long-term process. For individuals diagnosed with mental illnesses, the chronic state is a familiar experience. While the symptoms may fluctuate over time, or may be somewhat controlled by treatment, there is rarely an actual cure or final resolution of the sick role. When a person experiences a return to a "normal" state, the illness may be labeled "in remission" for a period of time.

In fact, for many individuals, the psychiatric diagnosis brings with it a professional expectation of life-long illness which will require treatment and cooperation for many years. Yet the long-term collaborative and mutually-respectful patient-doctor relationship with increasing amounts of patient responsibility characteristic of chronic physical illness is not the norm for those diagnosed with mental illness.

Although the current medical explanations of psychiatric illness are considered less stigmatizing than the character and moral defects attributed to "mental patients" in the past, the long-term treatment regimens for serious mental illness require the diagnosed individual to enter the sick role and, for all intents and purposes, never to leave it. Applying Parsons' sick role to psychiatry, the ideal obligations of mental patients would be to: (1) acknowledge their illness and seek help; (2) accept the psychiatric explanation for their personal experience; and (3) accept the psychiatric solutions, becoming a "good patient" for life.

In the model of treatment for chronic illness described above (Lidz et al. 1985; Charmaz 1991), recognition of the patient's experiential knowledge of the illness and self-determination in treatment decisions are essential to success. In a sense, the doctor is serving as consultant to the patient who is considered the expert in his or her continuing illness. In psychiatry, the patient's own experience of symptoms, life issues, medication effectiveness, and tolerance for unpleasant side effects is significant, and quite different from the experience of the treating physician or mental health staff. In fact, valuable information about such experience is only available to the professionals through patient self-report, and through behavioral observations. And yet, by the very definition of psychiatric illness, the patient's self-report may be considered less than reliable by the psychiatrist, particularly if self-knowledge conflicts with the physician's view of the situation.

Given physicians' suspicion or disregard of patient self-assertions, a process of redefinition is pursued. In this process, the more a patient complies with treatment and the more the patient's expressed reality concurs with the psychiatrist's understanding of the illness experience (which might be deemed "adequate insight"), the more the person with the diagnosis is considered to be a "good patient." It is expected that the more compliant a patient becomes, the more likely he or she is to improve, and compliance it-self can be seen as evidence of symptom reduction. However, despite this improvement, the psychiatric patient may not be expected to return to a normal social role and shed the sick role altogether, but rather to remain in a chronic diagnostic state.

An alignment of the patient's perceptions and condition with those of (normal) providers is one of the goals of any form of treatment, and a sig-nificant measure of improvement. In psychiatry, however, unlike treatment for some physical conditions, a patient is rarely considered to be "cured"—in fact, if symptoms resolve and the person feels back to "normal", the di-agnosis is ordinarily shifted to one where the illness still exists; it has merely shifted to a state called "in remission" which may continue for years. In this very important way, "mental illness" differs from both acute and chronic medical conditions of "physical" illness.

In modern psychiatry, a person who has been diagnosed with a seri-ous and persistent mental illness (SPMI) is rarely considered "cured" or completely free of illness. The implied expectation is that mental illnesses are chronic. They may remit but they are likely to recur. Compare, for ex-ample the yearly cold symptoms with congestion and cough that many peo-ple experience, followed by recovery to a "normal" state. In psychiatric illness, recovery from the symptoms would not be considered the end of the problem. The likelihood of a return to a symptomatic state, with resultant need for medical intervention, would be assumed. The comparable diagno-sis in this case would be rhinitis, or bronchitis, recurrent, "in remission." Next year, a person's next cold would be seen as a flare-up of ongoing, un-derlying illness, even if no symptoms had been present for many months.

For persons with a psychiatric diagnosis, especially for "serious and persistent mental illness," it is very difficult to return to normal no matter how well one is feeling. To the contrary, a former patient is always expected to become a future patient and the sick role is ongoing. In fact, if a patient believes otherwise, this can be considered a symptom of exacerbated illness; such "mistaken" beliefs put one at risk of intervention and further treat-ment. Once psychiatrized, always at risk: for illness, and for treatment.

## GOOD PATIENTS AND BAD PATIENTS

In the purview of psychiatry, a "good" patient is one who sees oneself as an ongoing candidate for return to illness (and to treatment), while the "bad patient" claims to be well. The good patient continues to inhabit the sick role, in a dependent or quasi-dependent state, while the bad patient resists the sick role and claims to know better. The psychiatrist maintains the power to define the situation, and the patient may be diagnosed with a psychiatric condition even when symptoms subside or are denied (with or without psychopharmacological treatment). The "chronic illness" adaptation of the physical sick role with its more empowered and self-reliant patient does not have a parallel in the world of psychiatry. The mental patient role, then, can be seen as a variant of the chronic sick role, without the pattern of increase in personal agency and decrease in medical authority, intervention and responsibility identified for chronic physical illness (Charmaz 1991; Lidz et al. 1985).

This disempowered role puts the psychiatric patient in an unusual situation. The more self-reliant a patient becomes, the more at risk for being judged ill or non-compliant with the long-term treatment cycle. (Keep in mind that we are dealing with what psychiatry calls "serious and persistent mental illness," not the so-called "worried well.") It is important to examine the ironic implications of a long-term dependency/sick role for psychiatric patients, with neither resolution nor power-sharing, and a continued recognition of psychiatric expertise even without a return to normal to resolve the sick role process. Under these circumstances, the problem continues to be located in the patient, who is defined as being unable to take responsibility for his or her own care. Success is then attributed to good care by the psychiatrist, while failure is attributed to a bad patient.

Yet there are important issues behind this comfortable (and far from benign) disequilibrium. By definition, if a person in the sick role is seen as having responsibility for the condition, or as avoiding treatment, then one's failure to meet the requirements of ordinary social roles is less readily excused. In addition, when the person resists the obligation to seek expert help and follow expert advice, then a more judgmental and less forgiving social response is likely.

When a bad patient resists seeking or accepting available help, actively denies having a problem, or is seen as responsible for the condition, then the attributions and reciprocal expectations of the sick role are transformed. The person defined as sick is seen to be maintaining the problem rather than working to solve it in socially acceptable ways. Only in rare situations is the sick role forced upon an individual. Non-compliant patients with diabetes, cardiovascular problems, or even HIV/AIDS, for instance, are rarely treated against their will. One exception is tuberculosis, which is defined as a public health problem.

In psychiatry, however, when voluntary entry into the sick role is not achieved, an active intrusion of social control may result, in which the person's state of disturbance or distress leads instead to persuasion or coercion by other members of society. Coercive and intensely persuasive or deceptive intervention, while uncommon in medical treatment, are routinely experienced in psychiatry. Ostensibly, the goal is to help the individual and help society at the same time by convincing or coercing the person to accept the help provided.

Goffman describes this helping process as the "betrayal funnel" (1961:140) in which a troubled (or troubling) individual is persuaded to accompany someone to a site, the case is presented, then the person is "sucked in" by subsequent events in which the power of choice is lost and others make the decisions through deception, forced choice or coercion. This entry into a "treatment" setting is not a voluntary entry into the sick role. To quote a slogan of the c/s/x movement, "If it isn't voluntary, it isn't treatment." Accounts of "betrayal funnel" experiences are common in the survivor narratives of the c/s/x movement.

## LABELING AND SECONDARY DEVIANCE

The defining framework of the sick role reveals its own limitations for understanding experiences of mental illness and the interplay of relations with psychiatry, the transforming self, and members of the larger society. The work of Thomas Scheff (1999) provides further theoretical explorations of these experiences within the sociological frameworks of deviance and labeling theory. As Scheff notes in his preface to the third edition of *Becoming Mentally Ill: A Sociological Theory,* "the theory in this book offers an alternative to the conventional psychiatric perspective" (1999:xiii). The origins, stickiness, and consequences of psychiatric labeling are important topics to activists in the c/s/x movement, many of whom use the term "label" when referring to psychiatric diagnosis.

According to Scheff, psychiatric labeling is a societal response to deviant behaviors observed within the context of social group. When a person persists in behaviors that Scheff calls "residual deviance" or "residual rule-breaking" (1999:53) (normative violations that cannot be normalized, "explained away" or excused as understandable "under the circumstances" by a person's family or peer group), an alternative explanation is needed for this behavior. Through societal reaction to the disturbing behavior, the person is labeled, stigmatized and assigned to a special status. The disturbing behaviors are seen differently when described as mental illness, and the person becomes a mental patient.

Scheff uses a set of propositions to describe the process of attribution and incorporation of the deviant role and the mental patient identity. In

Proposition 6, he describes how a person comes to accept the deviant role: "labeled deviants may be rewarded for playing the stereotyped deviant role. Ordinarily patients who display 'insight' are rewarded by psychiatrists and other personnel. That is, patients who manage to find evidence of 'their illness' in their past and present behavior, confirming the medical and societal diagnosis, receive benefits" (1999:86-87).

He takes the process further in Proposition 7: "Labeled deviants are punished when they attempt the return to conventional roles . . . Thus the former mental patient, although he is urged to rehabilitate himself in the community, usually finds himself discriminated against in seeking to return to his old status and on trying to find a new one in the occupational, marital, social, and other spheres" (1999:88). Succinctly stated, "Propositions 6 and 7, taken together, suggest that to a degree the labeled deviant is rewarded for deviating and punished for attempting to conform" (1999:89).

In Proposition 8, Scheff describes the next step of the process: "In the crisis occurring when a residual rule-breaker is publicly labeled, the deviant is highly suggestible and may accept the proffered role of the insane as the only alternative" (1999:89). The rule-breaker, having been socialized into same "role vocabulary" as others, becomes convinced and "begins to think of himself in terms of the stereotyped role of insanity . . . when a residual rule-breaker organizes his behavior within the framework of mental disorder, and when his organization is validated by others, particularly prestigeful others such as physicians, he is 'hooked' and will proceed on a career of chronic deviance" (1999:89).

Scheff quotes Edwin Lemert's concept of secondary deviation in explaining this process. "When a person begins to employ his deviant behavior or a role based upon it as a means of defense, attack, or adjustment to the overt and covert problems created by the consequent societal reaction, his deviation is secondary" (1999:72) (quoting Lemert:1951:76). This dynamic "deviance-amplifying system" becomes a self-reinforcing feedback loop, as follows: "the more the rule-breaker enters the role of the mentally ill, the more he is defined by others as mentally ill; but the more he is defined as mentally ill, the more fully he enters the role, and so on" (1999:94).

This theoretical approach is very appealing as a non-psychiatric explanation of becoming mentally ill. And yet, my own research question could not be answered by Scheff's propositions. What happens when this process does not work, and the person is not "fully socialized" into the deviant role of mental patient? The concept of secondary deviance seemed inadequate and somewhat simplistic after witnessing the complex experiential and diagnostic realities of psychiatrically-labeled individuals, and even becoming one myself.

Scheff's work concentrates on the labeling and the internalization process. He implies that the deviant labels conferred by experts and reinforced by the social group are fully internalized. In that case, are the complex identities of the former self simply replaced? Though labeling theory explained the attribution of stigmatized labels through societal reaction, the process of identity transformation appeared to end at exactly the point of "taking on" the deviant identity. The individual moved from one identity to another, accepting the deviant role assigned by society as a result of otherwise unexplainable "residual" deviant behaviors attributed to "mental illness." The social response of family, friends, and professionals created a coherent reality of explanation, a medicalized deviant identity that was then internalized by the individual.

The explanatory process ended there. It left no room for possible maintenance or revitalization of alternative identity patterns or role remnants, allowed no space for internalized conflict, questioning or challenge (at least, none that could not be redefined as "illness behavior"). Scheff did not go on to elaborate the process of internalization it assumed to occur. In particular, he did not account for a failure of the process, and the fact that some psychiatric patients, who had been defined as mentally ill in particularly persistent and ongoing ways, were actively resisting these societal attributions. The theory does not provide a means to account for the experience of these real-life "deviant" deviants.

In the revised edition of his book, Scheff critiqued his earlier theory [(1966)1984] for being "insufficiently detailed," noting that it was based on abstract concepts or "black boxes" and failed to specify "causal links between these concepts" (1999:158). His solution was to introduce the emotion of shame as a causal factor in the process of internalization. This causal factor may serve to strengthen his theory. He also recognized that "exclusion of personal characteristics of the rule-breaker from the analysis . . . probably limits the predictive power of the theory" (1999:196).

Perhaps, as Scheff realized, emotions and other personal characteristics are important in the analysis. These factors may influence whether or not the labels are internalized in the first place. Yet there is still no allowance in the theory for change that may occur in the rule-breaker over time, whether explained by internal or external factors, whether the change involves personal characteristics or expectations and opportunities in the environment. It seems that, in his effort to explain mental illness as an internalized social attribution, Scheff failed to account for differential response to that attribution. It was a totalizing model that seemed radical (since its "labeling" aspect could be used to deny the reality of the illness itself, but not the resulting identity), useful (to help us understand how people could internalize a social identity attributed by others) but inadequate (in its failure to elaborate subsequent developments and varieties of human experience).

The social contexts in which labeled individuals live their lives may be shaped or constrained in ways that encourage the internalized deviant identity to be dominant, and other identity aspects to stay submerged. In Scheff's model, the social expectations for deviant behavior bring the self-identity into line with the role expectations, and the deviant identity is confirmed. I propose in my work to go beyond that limiting point, to suggest that in contexts with different expectations and different opportunities, other (non-deviant) aspects of the identity and submerged personal strengths can and will re-emerge.

The clients I knew in the partial hospital program had demonstrated clear evidence that the internalization of secondary deviance and the assumption of the sick role were not permanent or complete identity transformations. This was true for people who were considered seriously and persistently mentally ill (SPMI) by psychiatric professionals, their families and support networks; it was even true for people who had accepted the medical model, considered themselves ill, and accepted many aspects of the patient role. Yet the literature of medical sociology and the sociology of mental health described above had little to offer in explanation or conjecture about the further movement in role development I had witnessed. These limitations brought me to the crux of my research problem and shaped the course of my investigations.

## ENCOUNTERS WITH RESISTANCE

In my earliest encounters with the psychiatric consumer/survivor/ex-patient movement, I met several individuals who been given a serious psychiatric diagnosis, yet were participating in society at levels quite similar to people who are considered normal. They often referred to the diagnosis as "labeling," and in fact questioned the need for psychiatric intervention and the appropriateness of psychiatric authority over those whose behavior was considered deviant by others in society and by professional experts.

There was variety among people who resisted psychiatric labeling. Some individuals returned to their doctors or hospitals for periodic crisis intervention, and others stayed as far as possible from the psychiatric establishment. Some worked in the mental health system as advocates for other patients or clients, and others advocated for a stronger voice in their own treatment. Some agitated for alternative treatments and/or the eradication of psychiatry, and others called for changes in the current mental health system to accommodate an increased voice for patients, clients, or "consumers." Some were on heavy doses of psychotropic medications that helped them to function from day to day, and others rejected even the idea of such intervention for their problems in living.

Despite the variation, they all had two important features in common: they were all psychiatrically diagnosed, and they were all "talking back" to psychiatry. Not content to settle into the sick role, or to depend on medical professionals to direct their care, they were active participants in selecting, directing or rejecting the care they thought they needed (or did not need). They were acting more like the patients with chronic medical conditions mentioned above: well-informed, active, speaking up about their needs, taking responsibility, and making choices about treatment.

## DEVIANT IDENTITY AS POLITICAL: ANSPACH AND BEYOND

In some, but not all cases, the rejection of treatment included a celebration of deviant identity. Anspach (1979) calls this "tertiary deviant identity," in which individuals move beyond internalized (secondary) deviant identity to take a position of ownership and redefine their identity on their own terms. "The politicization of the disabled represents an attempt to wrest definitional control of identity from 'normals'" (Anspach 1979:768). This model fits the activists I encountered. Anspach's typology of four "stratagems for stigma management" (1979:769) includes normalization, disassociation, retreatism, and political activism. "Unlike the normalizer," she states, "the activist relinquishes any claim to an acceptance which (s)he views as artificial and consciously repudiates prevailing societal values (1979:770)." She quotes the politicization of "articulate disabled activists" (1979:772) speaking out from the 1975 Conference on Human Rights and Psychiatric Oppression (see chapter 3) and the Mental Patients' Liberation Front, a group formed in Boston in the early years of the movement. By explaining their suffering as a result of social conditions rather than mental illness, these early radical activists legitimize their experience in a way that "allows them to sustain viable conceptions of self" (1979:772). This position also provides a link to social movement activism.

Anspach's analysis had a powerful impact on my thinking, but little else was available in the medical sociology literature to help me fill in the blanks. An especially important lacuna was the process by which people moved from the secondary deviant or "sick role" identity of "mental patient," with all that entails, to the tertiary phase in which the crazy identity was claimed, re-defined, and championed by its carriers. What would explain the differences I had encountered, variations that went beyond the deviant identity but were neither normalizing, withdrawing nor politicized? There is a gap in the liter-ature about people who fit neither end of a continuum of "mental patients" and "former mental patients." Yet there are many people who fall in between these categories, who create the spaces in between, who challenge us to un-derstand and characterize their experience.

The lack of explication of the transformation from a secondary identity to a tertiary one, even in their simplified essentializing forms, gave me the focus for my research. Sociology of medicine and mental health held few clues. Anspach (1979) never went beyond her original provocative paper on this question, and sociologists of health and mental health did not appear to respond to her ideas. Perhaps they hadn't seen examples that caused them to question further the assumptions of deviance and spoiled identity, and try to understand how real people could move beyond these stereotypical forms.

Goffman's work on stigma (1963) focused on management and infor-mation control of discredited and discreditable identities. He was writing before the era of liberation and identity movements and he assumed a uni-tary normative stance: "It can be assumed that a necessary condition for so-cial life is the sharing of a single set of normative expectations by all participants, the norms being sustained in part because of being incorpo-rated" (1963:128). An awareness of normative assumptions is essential to this research: whose assumptions, whose normative frameworks, are in conflict, and who decides what norms are to be applied?

Abdi Kusow (2004) has recently focused on current realities that chal-lenge this single-set normative framework. He describes the experience of Somalis who come to North America and do not accept the stigma of race, since it is not part of how they divide up their social world. For psychia-trized people to truly reject the stigma of psychiatric illness, they have to re-ject the stigma inherent in the illness or reject the illness itself. Alternatively, they can reject the notion that the illness is "who they are." These experi-ences are explored in my analysis of the c/s/x movement. Carrying out rad-ical identity politics requires an ability to reject and redefine some of the fundamental norms of society, which requires agency and the power to as-sert a claim to authority in the interpretation of experience.

## TALKING BACK: CHALLENGES TO EXPERT AUTHORITY

When patients talk back to their doctors, the standard hierarchy of doctor and patient roles is challenged. Rather than relying on the doctor's professional expertise and complying with treatment recommendations, the patient is exercising a degree of autonomy and personal authority that differs from the standard conception of a patient in the sick role. Renée Fox (1989) describes Parsons' characterization of the asymmetrical nature of role relations between doctors and patients as one in which the hierarchical relationship can change, but will not disappear, because of the "built-in superiority of the professional roles" (Fox 1989:25). Parsons relates this differential to a gap in competence between the professional and the patient, and the anxiety that patients experience, which makes them less capable of decision-making and more dependent on the doctor.

When there is a disagreement about the medical examination, procedures, diagnosis, or treatment, a number of outcomes can result. Power and influence can be used by both parties to negotiate an agreement or compromise (Gerhardt 1989). Alternatively, the patient can refuse to cooperate with treatment and consult another practitioner; a third option would be for the patient to refuse treatment and seek another alternative altogether.

These alternative behaviors are less unusual today as patients become more knowledgeable about health issues and available treatments, taking more responsibility for their bodies and the choices they make about their health care. The hierarchical balance has started to shift. The control of specialized knowledge by medical professionals and their role as gate-keepers to services still give them considerable power in the relationship. However, we have entered an age of commodified medical consumerism in which medical services are aggressively marketed, then chosen and purchased by more or less knowledgeable consumers who have differential access to resources, with intervention by managed care in decision-making about treatments.

Changes in the structures of service delivery are taking place in psychiatry as well as medicine. Managed care is proliferating, providing services to clients that range from Medicaid to Employee Assistance Programs. As control is shifted from the practitioner and redistributed to both the payer and the "consumer," through utilization review and "customer satisfaction" procedures, the relations of psychiatrists to their "patients" will also be changing.

## SELF-HELP ALTERNATIVES

The growth of self-help and peer support groups in medicine reflects the change in power relations between patient and practitioner, and also the power to define what counts as knowledge. Self-help groups have helped to fill the unmet needs of medical patients with chronic conditions like diabetes and cancer, who come together to share mutual support and the wisdom of their experiential knowledge, often by telling their stories (Maines 1991). Such knowledge cannot be provided by medical professionals, unless they share the illness experience. Self-help groups provide a further example of people with chronic illnesses who develop creative coping mechanisms for managing their own illness, with and without professional guidance.

Self-help groups have created a force that has brought changes to health delivery systems and a response to expressed needs of patients for more humane and holistic doctor-patient relations. This is a very successful model that has shifted the balance of power and changed the face of health care in recent decades. Thomasina Borkman (1999) describes it this way: "Situated within the voluntary and nonprofit organizations sector of American social-institutional life, self-help/mutual aid organizations function as consumer-controlled, adult-learning forums, peripheral to professionally run institutions, where the 'commons' space creates a distinctive agent of change through experiential-social learning" (1999:4).

Though the situation for psychiatric c/s/x activists differs significantly from standard self-help approaches, the literature of self-help provided important insights for my work with people in the psychiatric system. Borkman's earlier work (1984) had described the effectiveness of self-help groups in building social networks. In her more recent book (1999) she focuses on the importance of experiential learning in self-help settings. She describes the development of a "liberating meaning perspective":

> People with stigmatized conditions need a liberating meaning perspective that can free them of self-hate, a negative self-identity, and assumptions that they are inadequate. They need to redefine their humanity . . . A self-help/mutual aid commons exists in part to create a social space where people can freely define and evolve their own meanings and identity with regard to their shared problem, apart from the social groups or society that is devaluing them. From a societal standpoint, such commons can be incubators of social innovation and experimentation (1999:115-116).

It seemed a logical parallel to what I had seen in the development of a peer support group among psychiatric clients in the 1980s, and into the present. Borkman was writing in that chapter about a group of stutterers who were supporting each other and learning ways to cope, as well as improving their self-concepts in relation to the world of normals. Their group had been sponsored by a speech therapist Borkman characterizes as a "normal-smith": "an extremely open, self-help-friendly professional [who] from the beginning did not want the group to be dependent on him but appropriately coached the officers to develop necessary organizational skills" (1999:129). She cites John Lofland (1969), who "maintains that normal-smiths are critical to people who have been labeled undesirably different (or as social deviants), because the tendency in society is to assume that people cannot change: once a stutterer, always a stutterer" (1999:129). This statement powerfully reflects a clear divide with the more radical self-help position.

## A RADICAL SELF-HELP POSITION

Activists in the c/s/x movement support the principles behind self-help groups. Since the early years of the movement, providing opportunities for self-help and peer support groups has been a major focus. However, they reject the idea that a "normal-smith" professional, no matter how well-meaning and self-help friendly, might be necessary to appropriately coach a group of deviants into existence. It is useful to explore this difference.

C/s/x group members are not endeavoring to become normal. Peer-run groups provide an important alternative to psychiatric treatment as well as a locus for support and recruitment of new members into the movement. Consciousness-raising through sharing of stories, reframing, and politicization of personal experience into collective awareness has been enacted in c/s/x self-help and peer support groups all over the United States since the 1970s. Activists believe that they can help each other through mutual support, having a shared experience of oppression and rejection of professional authority.

As Borkman indicated, some support groups fail because they lack administrative or diplomatic skills. Yet there is evidence that professional involvement has also hampered their success. Self-help groups that have been funded by the mental health system, dependent on professionals for fiduciary services, have been denied access to their funds when their goals went beyond what professionals considered appropriate. The professional belief that psychiatric patients cannot change (once a mental patient, always a mental patient) also creates conflict over professional involvement in group formation. Even with the best intentions, it is hard to avoid patronage and paternalism when a normal or a mental health professional advises or sponsors a group (Freund 1993; Omark 1979).

It is also important to distinguish between c/s/x self-help or peer-support groups, and those run by twelve-step groups like Alcoholics Anonymous and Narcotics Anonymous. Unlike these groups, consumer/survivor groups are not designed to substitute a new fixed structure for their participants (Reinarman

1995). Rather, they may vary on a range from groups whose goal is to share experiential knowledge like more health-based groups, to groups that have a very political agenda and aim for consciousness-raising in the absence of mental health professionals. They do not share the official structure of a step-wise path or an official book, although the culture of the movement may indirectly impose a certain shape on participants' stories over time (Denzin 1990). Their goal is to create an alternative space and narrative that is separate from psychiatry, in which their stories can be shared and they can relate to and support each other on the basis of experiential knowledge about surviving the mental health system. The recognizable aspects of a "heroic survivor narrative" among movement participants will be discussed in chapter three.

## TALKING BACK AS CLAIMING VOICE

*Talking Back* by bell hooks (1989) provided an important key to my research and raised the question, what do black feminists and uppity mental patients have in common? A lot:

> To speak as an act of resistance is quite different than ordinary talk, or the personal confession that has no relation to coming into political awareness, to developing critical consciousness . . . it is easy for the marginal voice striving for a hearing to allow what is said to be overdetermined by the needs of that majority group who appears to be listening, to be tuned in. It becomes easy to speak about what that group wants to hear, to describe and define experience in a language compatible with existing images and ways of knowing, constructed within social frameworks that reinforce domination (hooks 1989:14).

Then hooks goes further to explain speech, power and the transformation of consciousness:

> To make the liberated voice, one must confront the issue of audience—we must know to whom we speak . . . writing my first book . . . I saw that . . . my words were written to explain, to placate, to appease. They contained the fear of speaking that often characterizes the way those in a lower position within a hierarchy address those in a higher position of authority . . . When I thought about audience—the way in which the language we choose to use declares who it is we place at the center of our discourse—I confronted my fear of placing myself and other black women at the speaking center. Writing this book was for me a radical gesture. It not only brought me face-to-face with this question of power, it forced me to resolve this question, to act, to find my voice, to become that subject who could place herself and those like her at the center of

feminist discourse. I was transformed in consciousness and being (hooks, 1989:15).

Reading hooks, I recognized in the c/s/x movement this same process of finding voice, speaking truth against power, finding that "speaking center," claiming authority to speak rather than be spoken for (or spoken about) without representation of your point of view. It was the role of the movement, of the "uppity mental patients," to find a voice to say, "It's not like that for us, you are not representing my experience, you are causing harm and claiming it to be help, 'for my own good.'"

There were strong parallels between what I saw in the movement and hooks' words. To speak against psychiatry and challenge its power from a lower position is a radical act. To redefine the relationship and challenge the hierarchy of power and knowledge is to place oneself as a subject rather than an object. To challenge the dominant discourse with a subordinate voice, claiming to bear its own truth, is a transformation of consciousness and being. It seemed that this was the right approach for understanding the c/s/x movement.

## VOICE, POWER AND KNOWLEDGE

Michel Foucault has explored many areas of power and knowledge: the history of madness (1965), the medical gaze (1975), the creation of expert knowledge categories from natural human experience (1978), the defining of acceptable discourse and practice (1970, 1979, 1994). All of these writings have informed my interests and my inquiry by raising issues of who has the right to claim the power to define truth and limit acceptable discourse.

In relation to the activities of the c/s/x movement, I was naïvely astonished by the ongoing disregard and discrediting of movement claims by those who "know better." The powerful knowers and definers of medicine and psychiatry held the power to define and influence both the expert and the public discourse, simply using their acknowledged role as experts to maintain the trust of the public. As Foucault describes it,

> Truth is a thing of this world: it is produced only by virtue of multiple forms of constraint. And it induces regular effects of power. Each society has its regime of truth, its "general politics" of truth—that is, the types of discourse it accepts and makes function as true; the mechanisms and instances that enable one to distinguish true and false statements; the means by which each is sanctioned; the techniques and procedures accorded value in the acquisition of truth; the status of those who are charged with saying what counts as true (Foucault 1994:131).

Meanwhile, I had witnessed the emergence of subjugated arenas of knowledge, of efforts by people to control their bodies and their minds, to define their own health and their needs. The knowledge of the psychiatrized was disqualified by the very forces of psychiatrization. The power relations that defined competing knowledges and claims to authority were an important part of the movement. It was more than a struggle against authority, it was about the control of knowledge that created the authority itself.

Foucault explains the special nature of this struggle:

> And in order to understand what power relations are about, perhaps we should investigate the forms of resistance and attempts made to dissociate these relations . . . It is not enough to say that these are anti-authority struggles; we must try to define more precisely what they have in common . . . For example, the medical profession is criticized not primarily because it is a profit-making concern but because it exercises an uncontrolled power over people's bodies, their health and their life and death . . . [These struggles] are an opposition to the effects of power linked with knowledge, competence, and qualification—struggles against the privileges of knowledge. But they are also an opposition against secrecy, deformation, and mystifying representations imposed on people (Foucault 1994:330).

In addition, the work of Foucault on knowledge emergence, insurrection, rupture and conflict can be seen in relation to James Scott's (1985, 1990) work on resistance and the "hidden transcripts" of oppressed groups. Scott's work reminded me of the undercurrents of dissenting voices I had known in the mental health system, where subversion and threat were suspected whenever patients were talking with one another. Dissenting voices can find each other, finding ways to speak to one another of and about their own experience. They can work to define their own experience, rather than simply being defined by the expert terminologies, to which they had no access as subjects, only as objects.

As Scott describes it:

> If the expression, "Speak truth to power" still has a utopian ring to it, even in modern democracies, this is surely because it is so rarely practiced. The dissembling of the weak in the face of power is hardly an occasion for surprise. It is ubiquitous. So ubiquitous, in fact, that it makes an appearance in many situations in which the sort of power being exercised stretches the ordinary meaning of power almost beyond recognition . . . Our circumspect behavior may also have a strategic dimension: this person to whom we misrepresent ourselves may be able to harm or help us in some way . . . With rare, but significant, excep-

tions the public performance of the subordinate will, out of prudence, fear and the desire to curry favor, be shaped to appeal to the expectations of the powerful (Scott 1990:1-2).

In Scott's characterization, the popular knowledge, the knowledge of the people, was shared furtively in spaces where expert ears did not hear them. And the expert knowledge was stolen to be used as a tool for understanding both the self and the expert other—to know about diagnosis and pharmacology not to define yourself, but to know the definers better and to enter into the activities of knowledge making and application. These are the processes of conscientization and liberatory education described by Paolo Freire in *Pedagogy of the Oppressed* ([1970]1994):

> As the situation becomes the object of their cognition, the naïve or magical perception which produced their fatalism gives way to perception which is able to perceive itself even as it perceives reality, and can thus be critically objective about that reality. A deepened consciousness of their situation leads people to apprehend that situation as an historical reality susceptible of transformation. Resignation gives way to the drive for transformation and inquiry (Freire 1994:66).

What a wonderful combination of tools, using Foucault (1965, 1970, 1975, 1978, 1979, 1994), Scott (1985, 1990), Freire (1994), even Clifford Geertz' (1983) notion of local knowledge to examine the maintenance, emergence, and liberatory reclamation of the silenced and resistant knowings of former mental patients. Foucault introduces subjugated knowledges this way:

> . . . there is something else to which we are witness, and which we might describe as an *insurrection of subjugated knowledges*. By subjugated knowledges I mean two things: on the one hand, I am referring to the historical contents that have been buried and disguised in a functionalist coherence or formal systemization . . . simply because only the historical contents allow us to rediscover the ruptural effects of conflict and struggle that the order imposed by functionalist or systematising thought is designed to mask (Foucault 1980:81-82).

With these words Foucault could be characterizing dissenting psychiatric knowledge(s) that have been set aside in the efforts to create a coherent scientific model of medical psychiatry. And the other sort of subjugated knowledges include a different kind of knowing, the experiential knowing of those with less acceptable expertise:

> On the other hand, I believe that by subjugated knowledges one should understand something else, something which in a sense is altogether

different, namely, a whole set of knowledges that have been disqualified as inadequate to the task or insufficiently elaborated: naïve knowledges, located low down on the hierarchy, beneath the required level of
cognition or scientificity (Foucault 1980:82).

In Foucault's view, it is the existence (and re-emergence) of the localized,
low-ranking subjugated knowledges that creates the potential for critique:

> I also believe that it is through the re-emergence of these low-ranking
> knowledges (such as that of the psychiatric patient, or the ill person, of
> the nurse, of the doctor—parallel and marginal as they are to the
> knowledge of medicine—that of the delinquent, etc.), and which in-
> volve what I would call a popular knowledge (*le savoir des gens*) though
> it is far from being a general commonsense knowledge, but is on the
> contrary a particular, local, regional knowledge, a differential knowl-
> edge incapable of unanimity and which owes its force only to the harsh-
> ness with which it is opposed by everything surrounding it—that it is
> through the re-appearance of this knowledge, of these local popular
> knowledges, these disqualified knowledges, that criticism performs its
> work (Foucault 1982:93).

Yet the discourse of psychiatry, despite the existence of dissenting voices,
continues to be a dominant force:

> in any society, there are manifold relations of power which permeate,
> characterize and constitute the social body, and these relations of power
> cannot themselves be established, consolidated nor implemented with-
> out the production, accumulation, circulation and functioning of a dis-
> course. There can be no possible exercise of power without a certain
> economy of discourses of truth which operates through and on the basis
> of this association. We are subjected to the production of truth through
> power and we cannot exercise power except through the production of
> truth (Foucault 1982:93).

Foucault describes the control and subjection, and Scott (1990) reminds us
of the residual, of the underside of power relations and speech, where the
alternative subjugated discourse is maintained in the form of "hidden transcripts":

> If subordinate discourse in the presence of the dominant is a public
> transcript, I shall use the term *hidden transcript* to characterize dis-
> course that takes place "offstage," beyond direct observation by pow-
> erholders. The hidden transcript is thus derivative in the sense that it
> consists of those offstage speeches, gestures, and practices that con-
> firm, contradict, or inflect what appears in the public transcript . . .

[T]he hidden transcript is produced for a different audience and under
different constraints of power than the public transcript. By assessing
the discrepancy *between* the hidden transcript and the public transcript
we may begin to judge the impact of domination on public discourse
(Scott 1990:4-5).

Describing not just a subjugated knowledge, but also a subordinate discourse, Scott goes beyond Foucault to bring in the relational element of resistance that always exists at some level. For human beings in the
psychiatric system, power relations exist in every interaction: when to
speak, what to speak, where to speak. In psychiatry, your speech defines
who you are, and it can be used against you. If you speak power's own truth
("shows good insight") then you will be free. If you insist on speaking your
own truth (limited insight, overvalued ideas, persecutory delusions), you
will be labeled and efforts will be made to cure you.

Scott describes the power of psychiatry to define reality in the face of
resistance:

The power to call a cabbage a rose and to make it stick in the public
sphere implies the power to do the opposite, to stigmatize activities or
persons that seem to call into question official realities . . . Rebels or rev-
olutionaries are labeled bandits, criminals, hooligans in a way that at-
tempts to divert attention from their political claims . . . Foucault has
shown with great force how, with the rise of the modern state, this
process is increasingly medicalized and made impersonal. Terms like *deviance, delinquency,* and *mental illness* appear to remove much of the
personal stigma from the labels but they can succeed, simultaneously, in
marginalizing resistance in the name of science (Scott 1990:55).

In Scott's description of social sites where hidden transcripts are maintained, it becomes clear that psychiatric subordination in hospitals is a perfect incubator. Even in the panopticon, there are places where surveillance
cannot reach. (Though as Goffman [1961] points out, sometimes other patients are not trustworthy and use insider knowledge to "reduce" their subordination.) When psychiatrized people have access to liminal spaces like
community drop-in centers, the talk becomes easier, while still circumspect.
Scott describes these conditions:

The social sites of the hidden transcript are those locations in which the
unspoken riposte, stifled anger, and bitten tongues created by relations
of domination find a vehement, full-throated expression. It follows that
the hidden transcript will be least inhibited when two conditions are
fulfilled: first, when it is voiced in a sequestered social site where the

control, surveillance, and repression of the dominant are least able to reach, and second, when this sequestered social milieu is composed entirely of close confidants who share similar experiences of domination. The initial condition is what allows subordinates to talk freely at all, while the second ensures that they have, in their common subordination, something to talk about (Scott 1990:120).

## SUBJECT/OBJECT RELATIONS

When a group of people are discredited precisely because they belong to a particular category, their point of view is not represented and may even be actively discounted or discredited. The dominant position of psychiatry, with its claims to scientific credibility in defining its human objects of study and practice, can be critiqued in much the way a feminist epistemology has been used to critique science. According to Dorothy Smith (1987), "The forms of thought, the means of expression, that we had available to us to formulate our experience were made or controlled by men. From that center women appeared as objects. In relation to men (of the ruling class) women's consciousness did not, and most probably generally still does not, appear as an autonomous source of knowledge, experience, relevance, and imagination" (Smith 1987:51).

Smith's point about women's autonomous knowledge, relevance, and appearance to men applies to mental patients as well. Paradoxically, the consciousness of mental patients is the focus of intense interest for psychiatry, but in a very particular way, from that center in which patients appear as objects. Patients' speech is useful in its function of presenting signs and symptoms of pathology in the psychiatrists' objects of treatment (that is the patients, or perhaps their illnesses). The patients' thoughts and experiences receive selective and filtered attention, interpreted in psychiatric terms for diagnostic purposes. As examples of utterances with their own autonomous value and relevance, with experiential knowledge, patients' words hold little credence.

To speak from difference and speak of difference, to claim knowledge and demand recognition, is to be further categorized. To be heard by psychiatry one must speak in the language of psychiatrists, reflecting their forms of thought, beliefs and values. This is a skill (a sort of dissimulation) learned by people labeled as mentally ill, a language they learn to speak in order to gain their freedom. To speak in one's own voice, in the voice that is only recognized as signs and symptoms, to ask them to hear that voice directly (that is, without psychiatric interpretation), is to lose the power one is trying to gain by speaking as an equal human being. The very act of speaking, then, is to be judged (grandiose, paranoid, oppositional). The power to define the discourse is clearly delineated and assigned, making it difficult to be heard without being defined.

Alternatively, Donna Haraway (1997) invites us to examine the power relations in technoscience, using the example of the patented Oncomouse® as an object of inquiry. In Haraway's view, as humans of biochemical makeup we are all implicated in the cyborg experience of biotechnology, being increasingly described and determined according to new knowledge variables. This being the case, we need to find new ways to negotiate the challenges of being positioned as subject or object in relation to scientific inquiry and medical practice. We need to enter the conversation and help to define it and shape it.

Members of the c/s/x movement resist the objectification described by Haraway. They are asking for recognition of their local, regional, experiential knowledge *as knowledge* and not only as data for the psychopharmaceutical research-industrial complex. Haraway makes this statement about point of view: "Technoscience should not be narrated or engaged only from the points of view of those called scientists and engineers. Technoscience is heterogeneous cultural practice that enlists its members in all of the ordinary and astonishing ways that anthropologists are now accustomed to describing in other domains of collective life" (Haraway 1997:50).

In a parallel statement, we could say that psychiatry, as a practice of technoscience, should not be narrated or engaged only from the points of view of those called psychiatrists. Psychiatry can also be seen as "heterogeneous cultural practice that [needs to] enlist" (and recognize) its "members" in this domain of collective life, not as objects but as subjects. With the efforts of the psychiatric consumer/survivor/ex-patient movement, the unrecognized standpoint of psychiatry's knowing/not heard, resisting/coerced object is being represented, shifted to the position of defining subject. C/s/x activists are asking for respect and recognition and rights protection—as fellow human beings, not as a special category of objects ("mental patients") who require "special" protections that can then be removed when their manipulation is deemed necessary for the purposes of "treatment" or research.

I do not want to imply in this discussion that the c/s/x activists, in moving from object to subject, would speak with only one voice. In fact, it is quite evident from my research that they do not. When a group is categorically discredited, the categorizing can create an artificial similarity ("mental patients") that hides the potential, and the importance, of recognizing differences among the occupants of such a marginalizing category. This is the kind of recognition that occurred for me in the day treatment center. And I have found that the range of differences, the variety of positions and experiences represented by the movement members, are what make the movement such a rich, lively, and hard-to-pin down area of study.

## A SOCIAL MOVEMENT

My first study of the c/s/x movement was a seminar paper that examined it as "a social movement" in sociological terms (Purinton 1993). In this paper, I analyzed the first year of the *Madness Network News (MNN),* an early newsletter of the c/s/x movement (described in chapter 3). The newsletter was first published in summer 1972 by a collective of psychiatric ex-patients and dissident mental health professionals (Hirsch et al. 1974) as an effort to bring the subjugated knowledge and hidden transcripts of psychiatric patients into the public discourse. The early content of *MNN* does not seem radical by the standards of other social movements. But as the breakout moment of this movement, the words spoken about patients' rights, against medication, against psychiatry, for alternative treatment—and in fact, the act of speaking itself—all this was very radical. The *MNN* provided a forum to challenge the status quo, speak the unspoken, and bring the hidden transcripts into the public sphere, blatantly challenging the dominant ideology by its very existence (Scott 1990). To claim discursive freedom for and by this silent (silenced) group was to reveal the possible, and invite participation of other silenced voices.

These are the beginnings of a social movement. As Bert Klandermans states, "individuals behave according to perceived reality" (Klandermans 1992:77). By disseminating information about treatment alternatives and alternative views of psychiatry, calling attention to human rights problems in the mental health system, the editors of *MNN* created a situation in which the personal gradually became political as the individual misfortune became seen as part of a collective grievance. It was not a sudden transformation, but a process of identification and growth, of building networks and calling for participation. Klandermans' definition of consensus mobilization seems appropriate here: "a deliberate attempt by a social actor to create consensus among a subset of the population" (1992:80). The preliminary stage involved generating a mood to participate, of making it possible to talk back, of winning "attitudinal and ideological support" for dissenting views (1992:80).

As more people voiced their dissatisfaction with psychiatry through *MNN*, there was a call from the editors for collective action by the readers; this was the next phase of talking back that transformed the *MNN* newsletter conversations into the "mad liberation" ex-patient movement. Alberto Melucci's (1989) concept of collective reality is useful in interpreting this process. Psychiatric survivors must first see themselves as a group, with shared views of their collective condition and shared goals and opinions, before they could come to the point of action. This was true for dissident professionals as well.

According to Doug McAdam's model of cognitive liberation as described by Klandermans (1992), consciousness is transformed through a process of (1) loss of legitimacy of the system (as the psychiatric legitimacy is being challenged by *MNN*); (2) beginning to demand change; (3) development of a sense of political efficacy. This model applies here, although I would insert a step between (1) and (2): the loss of legitimacy of the system was closely followed by a gain in legitimacy of the voices of dissenters, an important step of the process as described by Melucci (1989).

Over time, the movement reached a new level of critical consciousness. Ralph Turner's (1969) transformative model describes a change in which claims of misfortune become injustice, and petition moves to demand. Such a shift in the early c/s/x movement can be clearly seen. Awareness of injustice reached a point at which ex-patients demanded a right to decision-making, not only at a personal level about their own treatment, but at the societal level as well: demanding the correction of the social conditions that caused the injustice in the first place. For psychiatric patients this was a very heady transformation. From the early years of mad liberation to the present complex configuration, the c/s/x movement can be seen as a human rights movement in which the professional-patient power differential is challenged and newly self-aware "psychiatrized" persons demand more control over both their treatment and their lives.

## WRITINGS FROM THE MOVEMENT AND ITS INTERLOCUTORS

Most of what has been written about the movement is in the voices of activists themselves. Examples include Judi Chamberlin's *On Our Own: Patient-Controlled Alternatives to the Mental Health System* (1978); Irit Shimrat's *Call Me Crazy: Stories from the Mad Movement* (1997); Leonard Roy Frank's *The History of Shock Treatment* (1978); Howie the Harp and Sally Zinman's *Reaching Across: Mental Health Clients Helping Each Other* (1987); and Zinman, Harp and Su Budd's *Reaching Across II: Maintaining Our Roots/The Challenge of Growth* (1994); Rae Unzicker's "On My Own: A Personal Journey Through Madness and Re-Emergence"

(1989); Wendy Funk's *What Difference Does It Make? (The Journey of a Soul Survivor)* (1998); Daphne Scholinski's *The Last Time I Wore a Dress* (1997); and Kate Millett's *The Loony-Bin Trip* (1990). Edited compilations of consumer/survivor/ex-patient writings include *Shrink Resistant: The Struggle Against Psychiatry in Canada,* edited by Bonnie Burstow and Don Weitz (1988); *Madness Network News Reader* (Hirsch et al.1974); *Mad Pride: A Celebration of Mad Culture* (Curtis et al., 2000); *Beyond Bedlam* (Grobe 1995); Michael Susko's *Cry of the Invisible* (1991); *From the Ashes of Experience: Reflections on Madness, Survival and Growth* (Barker, Campbell et al.1999); and *Deprived of Our Humanity* (Martensson, 1998).

The literature of the movement exists largely as primary sources: books by activists, as well as publications like the *Madness Network News, Dendron News, The Key, The Tenet, Crazed Nation,* and *Labyrinth,* to name only a few; and the multitude of newsletters, flyers, poems, manifestos, and emails that I have collected over the past several years. The Internet is another important source of many movement-oriented websites and listservs. I am indebted to the many people who have been inspired to write about their experiences in the mental health system and their efforts to provide support, make change and fight for justice.

A few sociologists have examined this movement, including Phil Brown (1985), Robert Emerick (1989, 1990, 1991, 1995), Marie-Dianne Favreau (1999) and Caroline Kaufmann (1999). Allies in the mental health professions have also written about the movement, including Kathryn Church (1995), Maria Duerr (1996), Craig Newnes et al. (1999), Barbara Everett (2000), Lucy Johnstone (2000), and Liz Sayce (2000). Other allied professionals have written critiques of the mental health system and its practices, including Thomas Szasz (1970, 1974, 1989, 2001, 2002), Phyllis Chesler (1972), Peter Breggin (1991, 1997), Seth Farber (1993), Loren Mosher (1996, 1999, 2002), Michael McCubbin and David Cohen (1999), Breggin and Cohen (1999), and Terry Lynch (2001). All these works and more have been useful in providing a background for my research, and my realization that more investigation was needed.

Recently a new popular literature critiquing psychiatric practice has appeared (Levine 2001; Whitaker 2002a), written not by members of the movement or dissident mental health providers, but by journalists who have been in contact with the movement and have included its position in their critiques. At the same time, some psychiatrists have begun to attack the movement (Satel 2000; Torrey 1997, 2002) and its growing influence. The disability movement (for example Charlton 1998; Potok 2002) is also an important source for literature delineating the dynamics of the struggle for voice and alternatives to oppressive systems. This is all part of the conversation and I have learned much from its participants.

By incorporating writings beyond the sociology of mental health and deviance, I was able to see the issues of my research more clearly. The literatures of power, knowledge, voice, and action helped to frame the relations between psychiatrist and patient in new ways. The existence of the activist-advocate consumer/survivor/ex-patient in the mental health system, and a social movement that transformed these personal problems to public issues, began to make more sense.

Chapter Two

# Negotiating Activist and Researcher Roles: Methodological Considerations

## CHOICE OF RESEARCH METHODS

To learn about the resistant identities, beliefs and practices of people who are "talking back" to psychiatry, I used three different research methods to gather information about the activist experience. As noted in chapter one, this social movement has attracted scant attention in the sociological literature, from either the medical/mental health or social movement perspectives. To conduct this research, it was necessary to go to the source.

I approached the movement experience in three ways. The first was ethnographic fieldwork, or participant-observation. This method was used to gain perspectives and experience by entering as much as possible into the world of the consumer/survivor movement. (Sue Estroff, in *Making It Crazy: An Ethnography of Psychiatric Clients in an American Community* [1981] has written about some of the challenges she faced while doing ethnography with psychiatric clients. Mine were both similar and different.) The second approach was to conduct open-ended interviews with individuals who were active advocates in the mental health system. The interviews were designed to gain insight into their personal experiences of becoming mental patients and subsequently becoming advocates and activists. Finally, I collected and read both printed and electronic materials about consumer/survivor movement activities. These materials included recorded personal experiences of people who were active in the movement, as well as writings that represent and/or respond to movement activities in order to forward the agendas of the movement or its antagonists. Each of these

methods will be described in turn. In addition, this chapter will address issues that developed during the course of the research.

## INSTITUTIONAL REVIEW BOARD

*Gaining Approval*

Before beginning the field research or conducting interviews, it was necessary to gain approval from the university's Institutional Review Board
(IRB). This preliminary experience had an ongoing impact on the framing
and design of the research project. Ironically, some of the frustrations and
obstacles I encountered at the beginning of the IRB process (as a researcher
anxious to get started) were later reflected back in different (and more positive) ways as the research continued and came to a close.

   At the time of my application, the IRB had not yet created a separate
approval track for social science research projects. The approval process
was primarily designed for clinical research involving potentially harmful
and invasive bodily procedures. The challenge was to represent my research
project in a way that fulfilled the requirements of the IRB to protect subjects
from harm and protect their confidentiality, while protecting the institution
from lawsuits related to harm or breach of confidentiality.

   The proposed protocol for my project involved twelve to fifteen interviews of advocates and a separate application category for participant-observation. The participant-observation piece, according to IRB guidelines,
was approved as exempt from informed consent: as the subjects observed
were not to be identifiable in the research, the risks were considered negli-
gible. For the interview protocol, however, it was necessary to identify and
explain in my application any possible risks to the subjects; any potential
benefits of the research in regard to the research subjects, to the research
community, and to society in general; and also to specify how the confidentiality of the subjects and the collected data would be protected.

*A Special Population*

There was a complicating factor related to my defined "research population": it was marked in a primary sense by inclusion in the category of "psychiatric patients" both current and former. This group ("psychiatric
patients") raised a red flag with the IRB as a Special Subject Population of
mentally disabled persons, who are historically at risk for research abuses
and potential harm from participation as research subjects (as are other
groups including children and fetuses, prisoners, the elderly, the comatose,
and pregnant women). (University of Pittsburgh IRB Manual, Chapter six

Section 4, located at http://www.irb.pitt.edu/manual/chapter6.pdf) Therefore, in my application it was necessary to assure the IRB that the individuals I chose would not be current members of any high-risk group: they would be between eighteen and seventy years of age, not pregnant, and not considered mentally disabled (for instance, not institutionalized, clearly capable of giving consent) even though they were psychiatrically diagnosed and treated. In addition, the guidelines required me to assure my research subjects the right to stop the interview and/or withdraw from the study at any time, should they experience discomfort or impending harm during the process.

In the interview protocol, I chose to satisfy the IRB concerns about the psychiatric patient issue by interviewing only individuals who were presently working as advocates in the mental health system, so their capacity and competence would not be in question. In order to fit my research protocol, the individual had to (1) have been diagnosed with a "serious and persistent mental illness" (SPMI); (2) have subsequently entered into the deviant social status of "mental patient," assumed the appropriate "sick role" and received psychiatric treatment; and (3) be currently working in an advocacy role in a mental health agency setting. My interview guide included questions about their entry into the mental health system and patient role, about the experience of being a member of the community who was identified as a mental patient, and then about the experience of entering into the role of advocate for other people with psychiatric diagnoses as well as engaging in self-advocacy. Additional questions were asked about their awareness of, and relationship with, the larger social movement of consumer/survivor activism. As it turned out, almost all of these individuals were taking psychiatric medications and none were hospitalized at the time of the interview, though their circumstances changed from time to time during the years I knew them. As I learned subsequently, the categorical term "psychiatric patient" is constructed, fluid and more contestable than the IRB might have imagined.

### Other Ethical Issues

My project was approved after I fulfilled these requirements and was able to assure the IRB that my research subjects (and the institution) would not come to any harm as a result of my research. And yet the stories the interviewees told of their experiences of care and treatment in the mental health system revealed both psychic harms and physical injuries that led many of them to choose the term "survivor" to describe their ordeals. The ethical issues they revealed regarding both standard treatment and clinical trials with psychiatric subjects led me to wonder: Why were the relatively low risks of talking with me so carefully monitored, when so many psychiatric patients spoke about harmful experiences, both psychic and physical, that had occurred previously with no apparent protection and no means for redress? As I learned more about the ethics of informed consent, heard more stories, and worked closely with the members of this movement, I became more appreciative of the intent of the IRB process to protect individuals from harm, while I remained skeptical about its methods of achieving these goals.

Another aspect of the IRB experience has become more pertinent after the research than it was during the approval process. The ethics of protecting human subjects of participant-observation research, which raised so little concern during the approval of my protocol, present me now with the greatest challenge. After several years of ongoing fieldwork and participation in the movement, I am faced with the task of protecting both the activists who have shared their lives with me, and also protecting the movement itself from those who work persistently to undermine its efforts. My choices of how to speak about movement activities are guided by the following goals: (1) to enhance its recognition as a bona fide movement and (2) to protect its members' confidentiality as they have shared so much, while (3) contributing to the sociological literature by adequately representing the issues and activities that I have encountered, without betraying their trust. As the administrative requirements of the IRB process have marked both the beginning and the end of the research experience, it is useful to reflect on such issues through this lens.

## FIELDWORK: PARTICIPANT-OBSERVATION

### *Gaining Entry*

### *Background*

After successful negotiation of the IRB approval process, and before beginning the research process for either field work or interviews, it was necessary to gain entry into the world of consumer/survivor activism and mental health advocacy. Because of my previous employment as a social worker, I had some contacts in the mental health system. As described in chapter one, at a day treatment program providing services to people labeled as "chronically mentally ill," my colleagues and I had encouraged the development of a self-help group for clients in that program (Morrison 1995). Subsequently, the self-help group had grown to include other members of the community who were psychiatrically labeled; some group members had become more active, participating in the consumer/survivor movement at state and national levels. Through these contacts, I was already acquainted with a few members of the movement.

My previous involvement with this group taught me that mental patients and mental health clients could maintain a more complex identity than Scheff's (1999) concept of "internalized secondary deviance" would suggest. Although my contacts had dwindled in the intervening years, I knew these individuals were still out there, exercising their resistant identities in the community and helping other people to negotiate, challenge and reform the mental health system. I decided to become more involved in order to learn more about the goals, strategies and tactics of the movement as well as the experience of activism.

*Entering the Field*

I was fortunate to re-establish contact with one of these individuals during my first major field work effort. I had registered to attend the national yearly Alternatives conference in Orlando, Florida. It was essentially a cold entry into the field with no developed contacts. Before registering I had submitted a workshop proposal in which I planned to introduce the ideas of Paolo Freire ([1970] 1994) and explore how they could apply to empowerment in the consumer/survivor movement and in community drop-in centers. It was my goal to return some of my own knowledge to the movement, to make some sort of reciprocal contribution, and also to become more fully involved as a participant and observer. I was going there to teach a little, and mostly to learn about the movement. Fortunately this workshop proposal was accepted, and I registered to attend the three-day conference.

Upon arrival, I knew no one—but I could tell I was in the right place. The entire hotel lobby area was occupied by crowds of unusual individuals that I knew to be labeled as mental patients. The people in the lobby of the fancy hotel, checking in, smoking in the doorways, waiting in line to register, and playing cards at the tables and armchairs, looked familiar as I was very accustomed to being in an environment where people with psychiatric diagnoses were in the majority. Those who had registered wore standard conference tags with names and "Alternatives Conference" on the card inside the plastic case. It was quite an experience to see this group taking over the hotel, going into conference mode. In fact, it was unique and exciting and over time became exhilarating in a very powerful way. This particular conference was attended by over 1200 individuals from all over the U.S. (and Canada) and I was one of them, not sure what to expect in the next days, hours or even minutes.

As I lingered in the lobby as an observer, I saw the familiar face of a man (I'll call him Al) I had known during my time as a social worker, supporting the efforts of those who were experimenting with self-help. He called me over, we spoke, and it was clear that though he was pleased to see me, he was puzzled about my status and role in this environment. Why was I there? What were my intentions? We spoke at length and I explained to him that I was no longer a social worker but now a graduate student doing research on the movement; and also that I had, in the interim, myself been diagnosed and treated by psychiatry. In addition, I was there as a workshop presenter. As I was to learn, categorical status has an importance in the movement that can seem quite contradictory in its effects—first defining a person according to one's various labels, roles and history in the mental health system (the psychiatric consumer/survivor or professional identity) and/or the movement, and then being potentially redefined and over-ridden by one's goals, values, and commitment to the movement itself.

This combination of identities, and this moment of re-acquaintance on new terms, became the key to my entry into the movement. Al, who had been active in the national movement for years (something I had not previously known about him), began to introduce me to some key people who were there in the lobby. "This is Linda, I want you to meet her—I've known her for years. She wants to learn about our movement, she is a consumer, and she supported us when we were organizing in Pittsburgh. She's good people." The others respected Al and valued his opinion; they were friendly and welcoming to me, and gave me names and introductions to some of the important members of the group.

*Reflexive Aspects*

Reflecting back, I realize how pivotal this moment became in my research. It was clearly my point of entry into participation in the movement. Starting from this point, I was given access and trust due to his recommendation. They knew I was there as a researcher among my other identities. From there it was a chain of acceptance, and my gradually developing participation made possible a level of observation that would allow me to be a part of the movement. My participation provided important insights into the complex web of issues, identities, goals, strategies and tactics that make up the consumer/survivor/ex-patient movement. I believe these insights have been essential to gaining a deeper understanding of the movement and I will always be grateful for the trusting welcome I received in the lobby that afternoon.

As a person who had been diagnosed and treated by psychiatry, I found that it became increasingly comfortable to participate in these meetings.

Over time I became aware of my own experience as a participant and became more authentically involved through my own process of identity transformation. The main discomfort I felt was an interesting experience of questioning whether I was exploiting my own stigmatized identity by coming out as a former psychiatric patient, and whether I was authentic having never been hospitalized or shocked, treated against my will, or put in restraints. I experienced concern that I was not a genuine participant, that I was somehow exploiting others' experience for my own personal gain. Over time, I was able to discuss these concerns with some members of the movement who reassured me (1) that my acute concern was evidence enough for them of my good intentions, and (2) that my presence and involvement were just as valid as any other individual in attendance at the meetings. In the current mental health system, I was told, many people are never hospitalized but are still diagnostically labeled and still experience the power imbalance and challenges of psychiatric treatment and stigma.

At first I was seen (and saw myself) as one of "the wise" (Goffman 1963:19)—a sympathetic person who understood and was comfortable with the stigmatized group, as a former dissident provider and ally, but not a person who carried the stigmatized identity. As time went on, the movement themes began to resonate with my own experience with a psychiatric label, and with psychiatric treatment. I began to recognize and struggle with my own identity as a member of this group, though thankfully I had not suffered in the same way as many others. Through conversations with leading activists (like Judi Chamberlin and Kris Yates) I learned what it means to recognize one's affinity with the group, to internalize this identity and to be accepted as an insider by group members. I had moved from "wise ally" to participant.

### Field Experience: Movement Conferences and Meetings

Because the annual Alternatives conferences are the most visible public events of the movement, I chose to attend these major annual national conferences as a participant-observer. The Alternatives conferences are funded by the federal Center for Mental Health Services (one of the victories of the movement that has also led to some contention between factions). The politics of the movement dictate that each year the conference is hosted by a different organization in a different part of the country. These groups have historically developed competing philosophies (explored in chapter three) and the personalities of the leadership figures sometimes exhibit competition for loyalty and movement clout. So the conferences are good barometers of these competitive maneuverings, revealing shifts in power and affiliations reflected in the larger movement. I was able to observe and learn what topics, issues and approaches were addressed at these meetings; who attended (and who didn't); how they interacted; who was invited to speak; and what responses were demonstrated by those in attendance. Informal conversations revealed many aspects of what participation in these meetings meant to those who attended.

Over the next months and years I attended many more meetings at the regional and national levels: conferences of the state mental health consumer association, national Alternatives conferences, and annual meetings of the National Association for Rights Protection and Advocacy (NARPA). (See Appendix A for a list of conferences attended.) I participated fully in all these meetings—attending plenary sessions, meals, workshops, talent shows, and a protest demonstration at a state hospital in California; leading workshops, working at book and information tables, and helping with orientation groups for first-time attendees. The conferences were attended by hundreds of people who were self-identified as mental health consumers, activists, advocates, and survivors of psychiatry (some fit in multiple categories; the differences will be explored in chapter three.) Also present were smaller numbers of psychiatrists, mental health workers, and "family members," some of whom were also identified as consumers or survivors of psychiatric treatment.

Conference attendees participated in workshops, plenary sessions, special-interest caucuses, demonstrations, talent shows and skits, creative arts projects, and protest demonstrations. All these events focused on issues of (1) changing the mental health delivery system and the practice of psychiatry, (2) bypassing the mental health system and the practice of psychiatry, (3) harmful encounters with the mental health system and the practice of psychiatry, (4) empowering those who have received diagnoses and treatment from the mental health system and psychiatry, (5) protecting the rights of those who encounter the mental health system and psychiatric treatment, and (6) expanding and strengthening the local, national, and international network of the movement for human rights in psychiatry. The themes of meeting activities at the state level were similar to those at national meetings. They reflected concerns of the larger movement as well as ongoing local and regional issues and campaigns.

The conferences function as focal points for the movement. Each annual event (and there are several, since they are sponsored by different organizations) attracts new and old activists from around the U.S. and other nations. Scheduled workshops, trainings, caucuses, and plenary events focus on energizing the movement by bringing people together, providing new skills, reinforcing support and direction for movement activities, and building membership strength by emphasizing the history, goals, successes, and challenges met during the previous year. Closed caucus meetings bring together people with specific concerns such as survivors of ECT, seclusion and restraint, forced treatment, rape and incest; people of color, gays and lesbians, veterans, and other interest groups, providing a safe place to raise special-interest issues. Later, the caucuses report to the larger group.

In addition to the conferences, I attended three other historic meetings that were each differently designed to promote member involvement and infuse new energy and direction for the movement. Two were strategy meetings for movement leaders sponsored by Support Coalition International, which were held at the legendary Highlander Center in Tennessee. The third was a "National Summit of Mental Health Consumers" (sponsored by the Mental Health Consumers Self-Help Clearinghouse), in which activists from every state came together in Oregon to develop a series of "consensus planks" on important movement issues in an effort to create a national agenda and a national organization. Being a part of these meetings, by invitation in each case, led me to a much deeper and broader understanding of the movement, its history, its resources, its strongest leaders, and its future. I am privileged to be a witness to the energy and the dedication of these activists, and to be able to make my own contribution to this process.

My field observations afforded me the opportunity to observe the movement itself, public responses to its participants, and responses to its impact as well. By attending these meetings, and getting to know many of the activists over time, I was able to learn in depth about the issues and concerns of the movement, as well as the interpersonal rewards and support gained by participation and ongoing relationships. The conferences were total-immersion experiences in which the participants stayed in large hotels for a three to four day period: they spent time together eating meals, attending plenary sessions and workshops, enjoying informal break times, going on outings, etc. Aside from the intended content experiences of the meetings, as presented in the schedules of official activities, some important unintended interactive experiences should also be mentioned as significant.

## Relations with "Normals"

Often there was a unique "taking over from the normals" experience at the conference hotels: the ordinary business meetings, family vacations, and other activities that were going on at the hotel continued as usual, at the same time that most hotel guests could be identified as mental patients. This was often a very unusual experience, and it was especially revealing

to observe the responses of the apparent normals who perhaps had not encountered people diagnosed with serious mental illness before, and certainly not in massive numbers in a public hotel accommodation such as a
lobby or an elevator. These interactions were revealing in an "in-your-
face" kind of social movement, identity politics way—yes we are here, and
we share the world with you—we will not be ignored. To quote a movement slogan, "There are more of us than you think." In a setting where a
generally stigmatized group has been experiencing a powerful collective
identity and a dynamic of being in the majority, the interaction patterns
change and the experience of stigma is transformed to one of celebration
and ownership (Anspach 1979).

In addition, the relations with hotel staff were always interesting to
observe. At some conferences, particular concerns had been addressed be-
forehand. Staff might receive training from activists to sensitize them to
working with this population—overcoming their concerns, fears and mis-
conceptions. The challenge was especially high for wait staff in the ban-
quet rooms, serving guests who may be unaccustomed to such service
(staff worked exceedingly hard and were usually acknowledged and
thanked with great applause at the final plenary session meal), and for the
reception area staff who made the room arrangements, dealt with dissatisfactions and misunderstandings, etc. With each attendee-staff interaction, the staff members were learning something new about people who
had been identified as mentally ill. As an observer, I was able to appreciate and learn from these encounters. In addition, as a participant in the
conference, I myself was also viewed within the frame of the mentally ill
and could observe how people's expectations and responses of me were
shaped by their categorical thinking. I admit I sometimes felt discomfort
in this frame, but sometimes enjoyed the freedom of it, and often was
aware of the opportunity to reshape their thinking by being who I was,
and also a person with a psychiatric diagnosis. It was an interesting experience to say the least.

My experiences as participant-observer were enhanced by unexpected
contacts with movement members outside the meetings as well as within the
conference environment, and in observing interactions with the general
public. There were many opportunities to observe the negative public responses that provoke some of the motivations behind movement activism:
obvious disrespect, avoidance, insults, open staring and revulsion, as well as
simple curiosity. Children often were most honest about their curiosity,
while their accompanying adults often made efforts to disattend who and
what was all around them.

I encountered similar experiences on hotel-to-airport van transports, in airports, and in planes. At times, it seemed almost the entire gate area was filled with an unusual group of people, many in wheelchairs, who brought their community spirit into the public area with enough critical mass to change the tone and the experience for everyone. These experiences were a sort of carryover of the spirit of the meetings, bringing the movement into the community.

An interesting moment of transition often occurred between conference programs, as the hotel meeting rooms were being transferred from one conference to another, or as two conferences were being held in adjacent areas. On several occasions I was approached by professionals of various sorts who were attending their own conferences. These individuals asked curiously about the identity of our group: what kind of conference is this? It was interesting to be able to explain the existence, and the "conference-ability," of this group and its goals and grievances as a social movement. A conference of present and former mental patients? In every "cross-conference" interaction I experienced, the surprise and puzzlement of the inquirer was apparent. Such interactions were often discussed with humor and enthusiasm among movement participants; it was a chance to educate the public and fight traditional stigmatizing attitudes. Surprise is often a very effective tactic.

*Workshop Leader*

Another aspect of my participation was as workshop leader. I presented workshops on the methods and principles of Paolo Freire's (1994) "liberatory education" and on bioethical principles of informed consent. In this way, I was able to offer my own knowledge to make a contribution to the movement, and not just use the experience for my own personal benefit. In these small workshop groups, people have shared their experiences and their hopes and frustrations in very personal ways. As a workshop leader as well as participant, my experience of the movement has been enhanced through this give-and-take involvement, and my own participation has been authentic and engaged—emotionally, intellectually, and physically.

This participatory involvement has also led to a deeper understanding of the current and historical rifts, feuds, and splits of the movement. Individuals openly discussed their anger and frustration about the ongoing oppositions and resentments that have caused subgroups to work at times against each other and even against the success of the larger movement. Becoming aware of these issues as a result of trusting relationships has helped me to see the factors that affect movement loyalties and disturbances, at particular historical points and evolving over time.

*Behind the Book Table*

A final way in which my conference fieldwork enhanced my learning was through the "book table" experience. At my first conference, the group from Support Coalition International needed help staffing their book sales and information table and invited me to volunteer. Over time, I became a regular book table staffer. Through my hours behind the table, at that conference and subsequent ones, I met countless people (curious newcomers, recent activists, and the revered heroes of the movement), learned about movement activities all over the U.S. and the world, and became familiar with the literature of the movement, which I will discuss in the archival research section of this chapter.

*Field Experiences: Local Community Involvement*

*Making Contacts*

Besides attending national and regional conferences, I became actively involved in local-level activities promoting increased consumer representation in the mental health system. My local contacts from earlier work as a mental health therapist provided avenues for early contacts. Through those original contacts, I met more individuals who were working as advocates in the mental health system. For example, as the instructor for a sociology course on Mental Health and Illness, I invited two local activists to speak in my classroom. They spoke about their experience of the mental health system and about their personal and public advocacy efforts. The enthusiastic response of the students led to further contact with these individuals. I began attending meetings of local groups that were working to improve the responsiveness of the care system to the needs of its users. In this way I became actively involved in local advocacy activities where consumer voices were being raised and their concerns were being addressed.

*Attending Meetings*

I attended monthly Community Support Program meetings; other community meetings and public hearings related to reform of the mental health system; joined in efforts to organize a local support group and peer support center; helped to create dialogues between mental health practitioners and consumers; helped to organize a protest at a psychiatric conference on electroshock therapy. These field activities brought me into the community network of advocacy and activism. Active participation, and my multiply-identified status as researcher, consumer, and ally, brought me into contact with people at all levels of the mental health system. These activities also led to contacts for interviews with working advocates.

At first the emphasis was on observation. I paid close attention to the ways in which public and mental health officials, as well as other stakeholders in mental health services delivery, addressed and responded to both consumers and their issues in these meetings. I also watched closely how the consumers, who have just recently been allowed at the table (more on this in relation to opportunity structures, later), learned to use their voice in more or less effective ways. There are varying degrees of give-and-take in these policy and advocacy environments; over a period of several years now I have seen major changes take place, as well as resistance and entrenchment in some areas. In this way, I have seen the effects of the consumer movement in mental health (more on this word in chapters three and four) operating in a particular social and political context as it adjusts to major changes: these include a shift to managed care in delivery of public mental health services, and a major shift in political organization and authority.

Over time, I became less of a neutral observer and more of a participant. As I got to know the players, it was easier to get involved in the activity—to ask questions, to make points about how to respond to consumer needs, to raise issues that were being ignored or glossed over. It was quite an unusual experience to be identified as a consumer, and even an advocate, as well as a university academic and a former service provider.

## Consumer-Provider Dialogues

In another dimension of community work, I was involved in organizing and conducting dialogues to increase communication between providers (mostly psychiatric residents) and the recipients of services. These dialogues were intended to increase awareness of the recipients' points of view on the part of service providers. They also help the recipients to see their providers as human beings who are challenged with the responsibility for others' care. We hoped to increase communication and understanding of the different points of view, with an eye to a shift in power relations.

These dialogues had mixed results, though the doctors did report new insight into the concerns of their patients. One of the most important consequences, as with other community activities, has been a marked increase of confidence and voice for the consumer participants, and a strengthened group awareness among members of the consumer community. As a participant, I was able to observe the interactions before, during and after the dialogues over time. In this way I learned more about the issues, strengths, and challenges of activists' efforts to change the status quo in "mental health service delivery." Their efforts are often frustrated and gains are small.

## Ethical Issues of Fieldwork

The ambiguity of my position allowed access to many conversations and meetings that I might not otherwise have seen. At the same time, I was clear that I was engaged in dissertation research on the consumer/survivor movement, and I have served as a resource for the advocacy community. It was my personal involvement that made the research work possible, and it was the research work that led to the personal involvement. I was invited to serve on boards and committees of various organizations. (For instance, two boards of directors of consumer/survivor groups, and co-chair of a board that was forming a new consumer-run agency.) I declined in order to avoid potential conflicts of interest with my position as a researcher, and I was honest about expressing my reasoning.

I did not want to be placed in the position of obligation or loyalty to a particular group, without maintaining my freedom to criticize and keep a balanced view of the movement and its activities. I was always a free player, without allegiance to any particular group or agency, not on the payroll of any institution save my own university for teaching, research, and advising of undergraduates. I have served as a member of one community advisory board for a program that interviews service recipients about their satisfaction with services; I saw no potential conflict of interest in this community service.

## Emotions in Fieldwork

Over time, I learned a great deal as a result of the ambiguity of my role as consumer-activist-researcher-student. These multiple statuses gave me experiences that were extremely valuable in understanding the interactions between consumer/survivors, providers of services, and administrators and planners; between members, allies, and enemies of the movement as they negotiated and played out their roles for different purposes in so many different settings. My own shifting roles, and people's responses to them, brought me to experience many of the responses that are felt by people in the movement as they encounter the system—anger, frustration, joy, shock, relief, stubborn tenacity, purposeful manipulation—emotions and tactics that are well-known in the movement. I was able to share and reflect on these experiences with others, and I had to be constantly aware of my position and point of view in various interactions.

Unlike other activists, I could retreat to a more protected status, and to a life that was free of the influence of the mental health system. But these individuals lived and worked with the decisions and manipulations of the system every day; for them there was no escape. During stressful times, often created by the demands of the changing system, several activists were hospitalized as a result of increased personal suffering and psychiatric or physical symptoms. Each individual responded differently to the limited options that were available for help through painful times. These experiences provided more lessons about the movement and its goals—promoting the freedom to choose, and developing alternatives for community supports without losing choices through hospitalization and increased medication. This topic of hospitalization and advocacy will be further discussed in chapter four, as it relates to personal identity and the struggle for recognition, respect, and self-determination.

### Insider Status Issues

> One of the respects in which worlds, and various forms within the same world, differ from one another is how near or how far they bring objects to the individual.
>
> —Simmel 1971:xxxiv

### Distance

My close involvement with the movement, while it brought me much access to insider information, also had some drawbacks. Issues of distance were encountered during both the data gathering and the completion of this dissertation. These concerns will be discussed in this section.

During the research I held and acted from multiple statuses: as a person who had been defined and treated by psychiatry (psychiatrized), as a person who had treated psychiatric clients as a professional, and as a sociologist. Holding the viewpoints of all three positions simultaneously seems impossible, or it was for me, especially because they often conflict (see Kusow, 2003 for a discussion of such issues.) For instance, at a conference I could be caught up in the emotions of the moment as a panelist spoke of her experiences in a psychiatric hospital. I might be responding as a formerly psychiatrized person, feeling the emotions that were shared by the group in the intensity of the moment, and then remembering that I was a researcher and should be paying attention to the situation as well as my own feelings.

My experience as a former therapist helped me to talk with providers and understand their efforts to sympathize with c/s/x issues, and at the same time be frustrated at their inability to understand; meanwhile I could be trying to take note of the situation as a researcher. Sensitivity to these conflicts and contradictions developed over time and helped to reveal the competing views of a particular situation or position. It also became possible to consciously shift perspectives in a particular setting, taking various standpoints in turn, perhaps recognizing layers of reality as a result; and to create distance, holding back judgment and making the effort to use multiple perspectives, then to reflect on the experience.

Yet it has been a challenge. I am confident that my view of the situation of this social movement does contain considerable bias in favor of the activists. I have spent a lot of time on their side and I think their position needs to be heard. In effect, I believe that bias may be necessary in order to present their experience effectively. One of the goals of my research is to increase awareness of the movement and its issues. They are important and need to be heard, to be brought into the conversation about human rights as well as mental health treatment. The movement goal of breaking the silence is an impetus for this book.

At times when I spoke with other researchers they expressed concern about my bias in approaching the problems of the psychiatrized. They were probably right, from their own point of view. Indeed, that point of view has its own bias: an assumption of the correctness of the psychiatric stance. Research on psychiatric treatment usually includes an unspoken belief in the correctness of psychiatry. It may be examining the relative benefits of one treatment over another, but rarely questions the relevance or benefits of psychiatry "from a distance."

*Whose Side Are We On?*

The issue of partisanship is addressed in the debate about Howard Becker's article "Whose side are we on?" (Becker 1967) in which he states: "there is no position from which sociological research can be done that is not biased in one way or another" (1967:245). Hammersley objects to the radical interpretation "that sociologists are always partisan" (2000:91), but goes on to describe Becker's distinction between non-political and political situations, and how accusations of bias result. In non-political situations, the dominant view is not directly challenged. For this reason, "accusations of research bias are likely to come from superordinates, and will arise only when the social scientist does not conform to official views, for example by taking seriously the dissident perspectives of some subordinates" (Hammersley 2000:93). In political situations, with "subordinates being mobilized against superordinates, and their perspectives promoted," the credibility hierarchy is less clear. In this case, "accusations of bias can come from either or both sides, depending on the interpretations of the situation the sociologist adopts" (Hammersley 2000:93).

Hammersley's argument is very helpful in its effort to distinguish "accusations of bias" from bias itself. In any situation of political or power differences, the hierarchy of credibility comes into play. Clearly this is the case with the c/s/x movement's stance in relation to psychiatry, and vice versa. Further it would seem, according to Hammersley, the c/s/x movement's "coming to voice" during the history of the movement demonstrates its growth in moving from the "non-political" (totally disregarded) to the political (in actual contention) positions in this dichotomy (truly I think they are somewhere in between but still moving).

## Insider Status and Validity Issues

In acknowledging unresolved issues of biased standpoint in attempting to represent an unpopular position, I further hope that such issues have not resulted in the other sort of bias, that which threatens validity of findings. Insider status represents a disadvantage as well as a benefit in gathering, interpreting and presenting the data as a contribution to further knowledge and discussion of the subordinate position and its relationship to the superordinate. The results presented here do not represent all aspects of the movement, its supporters, and its detractors. And they do not represent the experience of all persons within the psychiatric purview. They are a preliminary effort to understand individual and collective resistance to the power of definition of persons by psychiatry as exemplified by the c/s/x movement.

## Insider Status and Disclosure Issues

The inherent bias of my insider position in the movement is further complicated by my participation in many meetings, communications and events over time, and the issue of continuous disclosure or lack of it. Although I was always forthcoming about my multiplicity of roles, and it was general knowledge that I was doing research on the c/s/x movement, there are undoubtedly people I encountered, or who encountered me, who did not know why I was there. And, indeed, often I was there as an activist as well as a researcher.

Julius Roth (1963) describes this experience when, as a tuberculosis patient, he began recording his experiences and observations of patients and staff. As a patient, he had a particular set of experiences at one institution, and a different set at another, with some overlap. His patient stance was obvious as he was in bed on the ward and treated like other patients.

His researcher stance was not revealed: "I did not confide my research interests or the fact that I was recording observations to any of the patients
or staff. They observed me writing frequently, but assumed that I was pur-
suing my academic studies" (1963:viii).

At the second hospital site, he discovered some benefits of sharing his
multiple roles with a doctor who had a lot to offer, precisely because she too
shared multiple points of view:

> Again I did not take any of my fellow patients into my confidence con-
> cerning my research interests. I did, however, tell my supervising physi-
> cian after I had been there several weeks, because she was a former
> tuberculosis patient and had much more knowledge and concern about
> the social and psychological condition of the hospitalized patient than
> one usually finds in a hospital staff member. Her support proved quite
> helpful. She called my attention to some ideas I had overlooked, espe-
> cially interpretations of staff relations from the staff point of view. She
> always encouraged me in my research, even when she realized that some
> of my conclusions disagreed with her own (1963:viii-ix).

Later he received grant funding from NIMH and "embarked on a new series
of observations of tuberculosis treatment, this time as a sociological observer" (1963:ix). It seems likely that his later observations were still informed by his former insider status, though he does not mention it. He
focuses instead on the methodological rigor of his observations. Later he
made the unusual move of asking for feedback from staff, patients and ex-patients on the initial draft of his manuscript. He found them useful for revi-
sion, though "they did not always agree with my interpretations" (1963:xiii).
I will discuss the issue of participant feedback below.

*The Activist Researcher Position*

My insider standing was my choice. It occurred as I was drawn into the belief systems and activities of the movement. I could have remained more
outside and I chose to move inside. I gained more access, and I made my
own impact on the movement as I participated in debate, strategizing, and
decision-making. This occurred at the strategy meetings, the national summit, the various conferences, and at local levels where I was active in the
Community Support Program monthly meetings, on the community advisory board at CART (Consumer Action and Response Team), in the
provider-consumer dialogues, and in the general efforts to create a more responsive and supportive community for people who were psychiatrized and
active in the mental health system as both workers and clients. I was not

being an observing scientist. I was influencing my own data by participating as an activist.

As an activist researcher, I was often torn between activism and research. Often I questioned the value of studying the movement and considered taking employment in activist jobs that became available. I discussed this with friends in the movement and they encouraged me to finish my research in order to help bring the movement, its claims and activities to the attention of the larger society. I was often conflicted about my choices.

## INTERVIEWS

### Recruitment of Subjects

Entry into the movement also affected my recruitment of interview subjects. IRB guidelines had suggested a formal and impersonal recruitment system involving either flyers posted in public places, or formal letters of introduction to local organizations where "my people" might be found. I chose to do things differently, with good results. Just as with the field research, I had no idea when I began my entry into the local community just how my early choices would lead to such rich discoveries and mutually supportive relationships with major advocates in the area.

It was the trust that developed through these community associations, and the acquaintances that were made, that led to my choice of interview participants. From my earliest proposal plans, I intended to interview between twelve and fifteen advocates who had moved from the patient role to an activist/advocacy role in the mental health system. My sampling technique was a combination of snowball and purposive sampling. I started with two personal recommendations (from two different sources), and these individuals introduced me to other advocates over several months of community involvement.

In this way my sample of potential interviewees expanded gradually. In my selection process, I chose to invite participation by individuals who represented a variety of ages, races, gender, length of time in movement, diagnostic categories, and experiences with types of treatment and hospitalization. Thus the purposive aspect of my choices ensured a variety of respondents with variations in life experience and experience with the mental health system. I stopped interviewing when I felt I had representative experiences, significant continuity of themes, and sufficient variation to assure recognition of differences.

I conducted twelve interviews over the course of the study. Each person recommended one or two others, who were chosen according to my perceived needs for purposive sampling. In order to protect confidentiality, I did not refer to other interviewees or mention which people I had interviewed. It is possible that they chose to speak with each other, but I assured all interviewees that their confidentiality would be respected. The interviews were audiotaped and transcribed. I analyzed the contents by hand, reading and re-reading in an effort to identify common themes, concepts and experiences that would shed light on the experiences of representative advocates and the movement in general. I also discovered counter-examples that helped to reveal some of the contradictions and discontinuities involved in this movement, and illuminate its complexities through the realities of individual experience.

All my interviewees were from the local area. Each person interviewed worked in the mental health system in an advocacy capacity. I defined advocacy as a position in which information and assistance were provided to enhance other individuals' abilities to negotiate the mental health system and to survive in the community. These were not positions in which any form of mental health treatment was provided. Advocates approach people in terms of direct problem-solving, empowerment and support, with a background of politicized awareness that mental health consumers face increased challenges and that's why their jobs are necessary. Beyond this, it is the c/s/x movement that has made their jobs possible, in a situation where being a consumer or survivor of the mental health system is actually part of the job description.

People contact advocates when they are being hospitalized against their will, when they are being refused treatment, when they are released from the hospital with nowhere to go, when their landlords are evicting them, when they need help applying for Supplemental Security Income (SSI) or other income supports, when they have problems with their employers, when they can't pay for their medications, when they want to go off their medications, when they wonder if their family members or friends need mental health services. These advocates serve as resources to mental health consumers and survivors in the local community, providing a special kind of service to people whose lives are affected by experiences with psychiatry and the mental health system, who are dealing with stigma and side effects, loss of resources, lack of information. They are a source of information, support, and understanding from people who have first-hand knowledge not only of the practical circumstances people face, but the discrediting stigma they have to overcome in dealing with the circumstances. In this way they provide an unusual resource. They accompany people to court, to the doctor, to other places where they need support and assistance in having their voice represented and their needs met.

One individual did advocacy on a volunteer basis; all others were paid full-time or part-time employees of local agencies in the community mental health system. All individuals interviewed had been diagnosed and treated (most were currently in treatment) for what psychiatry calls "serious and persistent mental illness," and all were willing to talk to me about their very private experiences, in tape-recorded interviews that lasted from two to three hours.

### Participation Issues

I was told by several individuals that they were willing to speak with me *only* because they knew me, or they knew of me, and were recommended to me by another advocate whom they trusted. I was also told that if I had followed the procedures recommended by my IRB committee (of posting notices or even sending a letter of introduction to their employer or center) none of them would have chosen to participate. I considered this quite significant.

Pittsburgh is a center of medical and psychiatric research, and some of my interviewees had been involved in research projects in the past. These individuals felt that they had been exploited in order to further the researchers' career goals, and were quite honest about expressing their feelings. I was told that talking to me was considered worthwhile because it was "for the movement," to "get the word out" about their own experiences and how they felt things should be changed. And they trusted me because they knew that I shared their goals and values and I was not using them for my own purposes. One asked me, "Why should I let someone make their PhD off of my suffering?" This tone of skepticism and distrust, growing from experiences of betrayal or disappointment, was a common theme during the interviews. This theme reflected an increased sense of empowerment and choice about what to get involved in, the freedom to refuse, and the freedom to make one's own judgments about relevant risks and benefits.

### Interview Content

The interviews were comprised of open-ended questions addressing several areas of experience. I asked interviewees about their experience of advocacy, both self-advocacy and advocacy for others. I asked them to describe what advocacy meant to them, how they became aware and involved in it, their goals for advocacy, and how they sought to achieve these goals in their everyday work. In addition, I asked them to describe their entry into the mental health system, their experience of diagnosis and treatment including hospitalizations and reentry into the community, their experience of stigma, their reflections about the appropriateness of their treatment in relation to their problems, and their relationships with treatment providers, family members, and other community members. Finally, I asked them about their relationship to and knowledge of the larger social movement, their views of its goals and possibilities, and their thoughts on the language issues in use of labeling or identity words such as consumer, survivor, and ex-patient. I also asked a set of standard demographic questions related to family, educational and occupational background.

### Demographics and Psychiatric Experience

The following is a summary of the demographics and psychiatric experiences of my twelve interviewees:

Seven women and five men were interviewed. Their age ranged from twenty-five to sixty-one, with a mean of forty-eight and a median of forty-nine years. Five were married, four single, and three were divorced, separated or widowed. Nine were white and three were African-American. Six identified as actively religious, with four Protestant, one Catholic and one Jewish. Six others also had been raised in religious homes, but were no longer actively religious.

Education ranged from one who stopped at eighth grade to two with master's degrees. Three had bachelor's degrees, five had some college training, and one had a high school diploma. Most had worked at multiple occupations over time, including sales, teaching, factory work, construction, paralegal, nurse's aide, clerical, and human services. Based on family history provided, six had grown up in a working class environment, and six in the middle class.

Their diagnostic histories had also varied over time. All had experienced treatment for "serious and persistent" mental illnesses, and most had been given a number of different diagnoses. These included seven who had been labeled with bipolar illness, eight with major depression, five with schizophrenia, and two with schizoaffective disorder. One also reported treatment for anxiety disorder, and several had experience with substance abuse. Three reported being told they had personality disorders.

All but one person interviewed was currently taking psychotropic medications ranging from antidepressants and anti-anxiety medications to antipsychotics, lithium, and antiseizure medications. Three individuals had experienced electroconvulsive treatment (ECT) (one reported over one hundred shock treatments). They reported a range of experience with restraints, seclusion, involuntary commitment, and involuntary treatment over their history of hospitalizations. These hospitalizations ranged from two to twenty in number, with the shortest stay reported at two weeks and the longest 121 days, except for three who had been institutionalized in state hospitals for longer periods. One individual reported a total length of hospitalization at approximately four years. All had also experienced community treatment including day treatment programs, outpatient programs, vocational rehabilitation, group and individual psychotherapy and activity programs.

Although four of the individuals (one-third of respondents) reported previous histories of involvement in activism (civil rights, labor organizing, religious activities), most did not consider themselves to have been activists until they began working with self-advocacy and advocacy for others in the mental health system. They reported that they were activated by their own experiences with mental health treatment and their desire to aid others in obtaining the care and services they deserved and found helpful.

## Interview Issues

I chose to interview individuals at the local (grassroots) level because I wanted to understand their experiences in a formative way, as they were evolving in the process of doing advocacy work in a local setting. While the movement has its "stars" and heroic personalities, it is largely made up of people working to create change in their communities at a personal level. My interview pool is limited by design, since the people I interviewed represent only a small group of advocates who are working in one county of one state.

While they are not a representative sample of all advocates who have been in psychiatric treatment and are working in the mental health system, their experiences with the movement and with the mental health system can be useful in providing an insightful representation of such individuals around the nation. Speaking both informally and at length with people from around the country, I have seen similar patterns and attitudes represented. Still, it may be true that my choice of (1) people who are employed by the mental health system and (2) people in only one fairly-conservative metropolitan area may be skewing the interview results toward the conservative end of the spectrum and may not be generalizable to describe the experience of advocates in general.

Movement leaders, and many long-term devoted activists, may have gradually shaped their experiences to fit the movement ideologies and narratives. Their stories are represented in written texts, tapes of plenary sessions, and movement folklore. Hearing from people whose focus is local, with varying degrees of influence from the larger movement, provides a sense of the ordinary activists who are working in the trenches of the mental health system every day, advocating for themselves and their peers in the community, and also feel connected with the larger movement. Their personal stories are also part of the movement. (In fact, there is now a concerted effort by the movement to gather and record individual experiences in a "Telling Our Stories" campaign being promoted by local groups all around the country as well as on several national and international websites.)

As part of my IRB-approved consent form, I made it clear that the interview was purely voluntary, and that they were free to withdraw at any time. I made specific mention of uncomfortable feelings that might arise in discussing past painful experiences, and stressed that if they should feel uncomfortable, they were free to stop the interview or change the subject. No one found it necessary to stop the interview. In fact, most individuals reported that they found it quite rewarding to review their own history in this way: to be asked to think about the changes they had made in their lives, and how they were working to improve the lives of others as well.

As is often true for ethnographically-supported interview research, I found myself thankful that I spent some time in the field before conducting the interviews. I believe the questions I asked, while similar to those proposed in the original research plan, were significantly informed by the field research in a way that made them much more pertinent to the experience of patienthood and advocacy itself, and also to the experience of the movement—across the entire range of awareness of movement activities. As my understanding of the movement grew, especially the complexity of its participants and goals, I was better able to recognize and appreciate the variation of attitudes and approaches that people took to their advocacy activities, as well as the underlying similarities.

This variation taught me an important lesson through my interviews. Early in the research, I had a rather simplistic view of what it meant to be an advocate and activist in the consumer/survivor/ex-patient movement: I was somewhat blinded by my own expectations of radical advocacy. As I learned more about the different attitudes toward psychiatry, medication and peer-support philosophies that were represented in the larger movement, I was also able to appreciate the differences represented in my interviewees' approaches to advocacy. In this way the individuals I interviewed enlarged my understanding of the movement's diversity of voices and its underlying philosophy of respect for individual needs and choices.

This is more than a movement of anti-psychiatry activists; it is a movement of people who are working to win human rights, respect and recognition for people who have been psychiatrically labeled. Many activists are using psychiatry and its treatments to help them to get along in the normal world, yet they actively challenge professional assumptions about who knows what is best for them, and subvert the expert "wisdom" about how and whether "consumer/survivors" will go about getting what they need from both the system and each other. They do this in their advocacy work, for themselves and for others.

Some advocates choose to live and practice the movement's principles and goals in a quiet, one-on-one way; others get more involved and represent their (individual and collective) interests by serving on committees and speaking at public policy forums. Some are extensively involved at regional, state and national levels. All have been touched by the movement, as the centers in which they work were founded and funded by its efforts. More or less focused on the larger movement, all have been influenced through the network of its individual members through trainings, personal bonds, or inspiration.

Each individual makes personal choices about activist practice based on individual capacities and talents, strengths and weaknesses. These abilities and commitments vary over time and circumstance as well. The interviews showed that throughout these variations in their activism and advocacy styles, their concerns and experiences reflect those of the larger movement. Relating these interview findings to my knowledge of the larger movement has brought me a deeper understanding of the human rights aspects which are deeply felt by so many individuals, all of whom find various ways to enact them in their own lives and in the lives of others, while supporting each other in their efforts.

## ARCHIVAL INFORMATION INCLUDING INTERNET

The third and final aspect of this research has been an effort to gather and study the archival and "artifactual" sources of the movement. These sources of information have included books, journal and magazine articles, government documents, newspaper articles, brochures and newsletters, videotapes, audiotapes, conference materials, announcements, flyers, poetry, bumper stickers, buttons, t-shirts, websites, email newsletters and alerts, and Internet discussion groups. Though I have by no means seen all there is to be seen about the movement, many sources have been available and I have collected many artifacts and documents. Some sources are written by and for the movement; others (far fewer) are written about the movement by outside observers and/or critics. Authorized tapes of conference events and transcripts of speeches have also been included as sources of data in the analysis.

These sources exemplify a wide range of representations of experience, strategies for change, and calls for action. Many voices are represented in these materials; their variety and persistence are what has kept the movement alive for thirty years, and keeps it changing in response to new opportunities and challenges over the years. Some archival material also demonstrates the impact of the movement, as professional practice and research groups have responded to calls for inclusion and consideration of "consumer views" in planning and practice of treatment and research.

## DERIVING THEMES

Exposure to the movement through fieldwork and archival research, and personal immersion in movement activities, provided a strong framework of movement beliefs and values. Yet it was the interviews that brought me to my senses in deriving the themes that would help to answer my research questions. The advocates I interviewed were a varied lot; only a few had chosen the drama of extensive involvement in the larger movement. Their entries into the psychiatric world were all different and their views of treatment also varied. Some were much more conservative than I had imagined. Yet all were dedicating themselves to advocacy and empowerment for themselves and their peers, based on movement principles and connected to its personal and organizational network.

Reading the interviews, over and over, I began to notice commonalities that were not so evident on the surface. The resistance that emerged was not always spoken, but sometimes came out in a more attitudinal way: a small remark, a twist of understated humor. Over time I began to see that the dichotomized anti-psychiatry or self-help framework of previous writers, and of some movement activists themselves, was blurring my vision. These individuals were not anti-psychiatry per se; they were resisting the imposition of definitions and constraints on their lives, even if they agreed with the definitions themselves.

The themes of the movement seemed clear at first, but multiple. I had yet to recognize the themes that sat at the core of the many goals I had noticed. Analysis of some "heroic" survival narratives for a conference paper helped me to see the process of help-seeking and betrayal at a larger level, which could also be recognized "in small." The little insults, the lack of recognition, the objectification, were shaping the response of these ordinary advocates that few would consider heroic. It was the resonance of these emerging messages with the louder themes of the bigger stories that helped me to recognize the fundamental, underlying issues.

Extracting quotes, separate from surrounding text, helped me to see more clearly the meanings expressed in the words. Recognizing emotions was a powerful part of the analysis, and they deserve further analysis. They helped me to see the forms of resistance (elaborated in chapter four) as responses to the unmet expectations of the steps in help-seeking and phases of development of resistant identity. Seeing the phases helped me to recognize the source of differences as well as similarities.

My interviewees were located at different levels of resistance. For instance, politicization in a larger movement sense is not an automatic response to discrediting and dehumanization, or even to solidarity and activism. Their ways of talking back were not the same. The themes are related to a form of survivor narrative and develop differently according to individual experience and core beliefs. The complexity of the movement is embodied by these willing people who cared enough about the movement to allow my interviews. Their own unique identities, maintained in spite of psychiatric labeling, allowed me to discover the commonalities behind this complex and shifting identity framework.

In the next chapter, I introduce the historical background of the movement. A complete history of the movement has not yet been written. This brief overview will focus on the origins and themes of talking back, and some evolving processes shaped by the players in their more recent historical context.

Chapter Three

# The Consumer/Survivor/Ex-Patient Movement: Historical Background and Themes

> Our history is out there. Our history is as important as the black civil rights movement, the women's movement, all liberation struggles. Our history will be recorded and written by *us*.
> —Judi Chamberlin, Alternatives Conference, Nashville 1999.

## OVERVIEW OF THE CONSUMER/SURVIVOR/EX-PATIENT (C/S/X) MOVEMENT

The social movement of "the mad" has been variously referred to as the "mad liberation," "anti-psychiatry," "psychiatric survivor," "ex-patient," "ex-inmate," and "mental health consumer" movement. The variety of terms illustrates the diversity of concerns, attitudes, and foci that have developed as the movement has grown and changed. Some segments of the movement have been extremely radical and separatist, working to abolish the powers of psychiatry. Other segments have taken a more collaborative route, working to reform the mental health system and provide more responsive, client-driven services and policy changes. Often they have met in the middle.

The c/s/x movement is not a centralized national movement with well-defined leadership, membership, goals and objectives. It has no official leaders, no official hierarchy, and no ongoing organizational structure. Rather, it exists as a loose coalition of advocacy and activist groups whose members engage in numerous activities designed to promote mutual support, rights protection, alternatives, advocacy, and information flow that will enhance empowerment and choice for people whose lives have been affected by psychiatry.

These movement groups represent a range of approaches to the problems people have encountered. They are local, regional, national, and even international in scope. Their diversity both exemplifies and helps to explain the coalition-style structures that have evolved continually through the movement's history. The wide range of needs and approaches personified by movement structures exists, and is maintained, through a particular emphasis on self-determination and recognition of different needs and concerns in the population it represents.

Over its history, the c/s/x movement has focused on several core claims in regard to people who have been labeled and treated by psychiatry (psychiatrized). The movement claims that: (1) psychiatrized individuals must have an authorized voice in their treatment and the system of care; (2) they must have access to information and knowledge related to treatment decisions, legal rights, and other issues; (3) they must have protection of their right to freedom from harm; (4) they must have the power of self-determination; and (5) they must have access to choice in their treatment and their lives. In summary, the c/s/x movement claims that psychiatrized persons should have the same rights as any other human being. The fact that the movement's members have taken different routes in advancing these claims illustrates that it is in fact a grassroots movement that responds to local issues and needs, to the vagaries of politics and resources, to the quirks and passions of its members, and the pressures of human experience. Like any social movement, its path is influenced by those who choose to create and follow it, as well as those who respond with support or enmity.

This chapter will focus on the origins of the c/s/x movement with particular emphasis on the aspects related to the history and development of "talking back" to psychiatry, of finding voice and using its power to work for change. Chapter four will focus on the individual and collective experience of voice, and what this means for the larger movement. Chapter five will characterize the larger membership and present some of the specific initiatives and campaigns that show the movement "in action" and how it endeavors to make change in the larger context.

## INTRODUCTION TO THEMES

Movement history reveals a continuity of two major themes: Breaking the Silence and Ending Psychiatric Oppression. Each theme incorporates major movement goals. I will provide a general overview of each theme and the goals it encompasses, then describe how the themes are played out in different historical circumstances, from the movement's precursors through four stages to the present.

### Theme One: Breaking the Silence

This theme includes two goals that have been emphasized in the movement's literature and actions throughout its history. Breaking the silence works in two directions: gaining voice to speak about the experience of psychiatric treatment, and gaining access to the information and expert knowledge that have defined and constrained that experience.

#### Gaining Voice

One of the movement's major goals is to provide a forum for the voices of people in the mental health system (psychiatrized people) to be heard. The emphasis is on the freedom to speak, to express the truth of one's experience with psychiatry, not to be silenced or spoken for by others. With the expression of voice, the next step is to create linkages for consciousness-raising, mutual support and information flow. The movement provides free space for individual voices and collective voices to be raised, to each other and to the world. Joining individual voices supports the collective ability to speak truth to power.

#### Access to Knowledge

Another goal, which is attained through achievement of voice, is to expose psychiatric practice to the light of day (breaking down the walls). Access to knowledge requires the right of entry to the expert knowledge of psychiatric practice. This includes information about the realities of diagnosis and treatment, previously mystified and controlled by the experts, which is necessary for informed choice and voice. It also includes access to knowledge about legal rights and alternatives.

Access to knowledge also refers to exposing abuses related to incarceration and forced treatment, revealed through narratives of personal experience. This knowledge is important to people inside and outside the system. Its exposure creates a power shift when abusive practice is shared by its victims and reaches public attention as well.

Breaking the silence is thus achieved through creating access to these hidden knowledges, combined with the interactive experience of silenced individuals coming to voice and sharing stories. The process can be theoretically characterized as an emergence of subjugated knowledge through provision of safe spaces, and an exposure of the hidden transcripts of the silenced and oppressed. This combined emergence leads to consciousness-raising, through which the movement begins to build a collective identity. Private problems are reinterpreted into public issues and participants gather strength to talk back to the power of psychiatry and the mental health system which has silenced them and controlled access to information in the past.

### Theme Two: Ending Psychiatric Oppressions

The theme of Ending Psychiatric Oppression incorporates three important goals that are emphasized in the movement's activities and literature. Protecting and expanding legal rights, claiming the power of autonomy and self-determination, and expanding the choices available for treatment and support have been central goals throughout its history.

### Rights

A major goal of the movement is to end psychiatric oppression by fighting for human rights in the mental health system. This struggle includes freedom from abuse, freedom from forced and harmful treatment, and the right to self-determination for people in the mental health system. The protection and expansion of rights have both been important, with efforts to introduce and enforce laws that protect the rights of people to receive psychiatric treatment (as opposed to warehousing in institutions) and also to protect people from receiving unwanted treatment through coercive means.

The importance of being informed about legal rights is also emphasized. This includes rights relating to mental health treatment and also rights in the larger community, including voting rights, rights in the workplace, etc. Advocacy emphasizes both creating rights and improving communication in order to protect those rights. Awareness of injustice and active efforts to attain justice are fundamental goals of the movement. They also provide a powerful sense of grievance and solidarity in building collective awareness and strength for the movement and its members.

### Power

Ending psychiatric oppression also means asserting power by challenging psychiatry's authority to define the needs and realities of people in treatment. Emphasizing the valued experiential knowledge of individuals who are defined and controlled by psychiatric labeling and treatment practices (psychiatrized), along with exposing and demystifying the expert knowledge claims, make the power of psychiatry more vulnerable to challenge. Challenging expert knowledge claims in the clinical setting, in the media, and in the public forum are all part of the c/s/x movement. The two competing narratives (psychiatric and psychiatrized) can then be compared in the light of day.

## Choice

The c/s/x movement has also challenged psychiatry by working to provide alternatives to psychiatric treatment. These alternatives are based on people's own expressed needs and underlying strengths, as well as the strength of the c/s/x community itself. With self-help and peer support at its base, the goal is to create a competing system of supports and opportunities to meet people's needs, based on their ability to help themselves and help each other with their emotional difficulties. This goal involves an ongoing struggle for funding, and efforts to influence policy at local, state, and national (even international) levels.

## Intertwining Historical Themes

The two themes outlined above have different emphases, but they are inextricably intertwined; indeed, their essential interplay colors the history of the movement. Voice is needed to fight oppression, while overcoming oppression is necessary to gain voice. Claiming voice and overcoming oppression bring a measure of self-determination and choice. Coming together in collective voice brings more power to create change, while personal differences and historical contexts of thought, knowledge and practice will shape available opportunities.

Divergent interests developed within these contexts have shaped the movement's expressions of its goals and claims, leading to different emphases among its members. This difference has led to the previous characterization by Emerick (1989, 1990, 1995) and Kaufmann (1999) of movement activism as focusing "either" on self-help (consumer, moderate, partnership model) or anti-psychiatry (survivor, radical separatist) issues. This is a dichotomy which I hope to dispel by showing the underlying themes and goals to be continuous in "both" segments of the movement, driving its underlying activism even when the emphases appear to differ on the surface. The history of the movement reflects these evolving tensions and efforts at resolution, while revealing the diversity of its voices, their claims, and their efforts at reaching movement goals in various ways.

When reality is defined and constrained by a powerful other who claims to know what you need, the need to gain voice is paramount. Even well-intentioned helpers, who speak for you without knowing your reality, will likely define it in terms of their own interests. Benevolent oppressors who are willing to "give" you power can later decide to take it away. In effect, power must be "taken" with awareness in order for authentic empowerment to be truly gained. Freire (1994) describes the situation this way:

> It is only when the oppressed find the oppressor out and become involved in the organized struggle for their liberation that they begin to believe in themselves. . . . Attempting to liberate the oppressed without their reflective participation in the act of liberation is to treat them as objects which must be saved from a burning building (Freire 1994:47).

In order for those who have experienced the strong definitions and controls of psychiatry ("the psychiatrized") to gain empowerment, at both individual and collective levels, psychiatric authority and expertise must be continually challenged. Voice, empowerment, choice and freedom are intricately linked in an ongoing effort. Perseverance and small victories are central to this movement.

The common experience of overcoming oppression and betrayal, explored in chapter four, maintains a powerful link among members of the c/s/x movement and drives its underlying themes. At its deepest levels, this is what I mean by talking back. Throughout the history of the movement, the themes have been enacted in various ways, and conflicting approaches have sometimes challenged the members and their interests. Yet the common origins of movement identity (the core unity of having been psychiatrized, the shared knowledge of psychiatric oppression) help to build unity against serious challenges in the fight to maintain voice, choice and human rights in the mental health system.

## FOUR HISTORICAL STAGES OF THE MOVEMENT: AN INTRODUCTION

The history of the consumer/survivor/ex-patient movement in the United States can be divided into four main stages. The Early Years include the activities of the 1970s, when the movement began. The Middle Years evolved in the decade of the 1980s, when the movement achieved recognition and was partially co-opted and institutionalized. The Recent Years correspond to the 1990s, when the Americans with Disabilities Act redefined the playing field and radical challenges were launched in response to psychiatry's "Decade of the Brain." The Emerging Years can be projected into the new era of the 21st century, as coalitions form and old wounds heal in response to increased threats and oppression from the enemies of the movement.

After brief mention of two movement precursors, each of these stages will be described in turn. Special attention will be paid to the earliest years, when core themes were developed and the movement's major voices emerged.

## MOVEMENT PRECURSORS: PACKARD AND BEERS

Historical precursors to the consumer/survivor/ex-patient movement are useful in creating comparisons with the movement of the present day. Similarities and differences can be found in the writings of Elizabeth H. Packard (1868; 1873) and Clifford W. Beers (1908). These two individuals responded to the injustices they experienced during their incarceration in mental institutions and worked ardently for reform. Their articulate and energetic campaigns were influential in instigating early efforts to expose inhumane treatment conditions for people diagnosed with mental illness. They called attention to the importance of treating mental patients as human beings who deserved respect and protection of their rights. And yet their stories also carry opposing themes which shed light on some of the differences shaping the c/s/x movement today.

Elizabeth Packard is an important figure in the history of activism in the mental health system. A minister's wife, she was institutionalized against her will in the 1860s and became a champion of rights activism for psychiatric inmates. Historian Gerald Grob describes her experience:

> The most spectacular attack on legal incarceration came from Elizabeth Ware Packard, who challenged both the subordination of women to their husbands and a male political and psychiatric establishment. . . When Packard refused to play the role of an obedient wife and expressed religious ideas bordering on mysticism, her husband had her committed in 1860 to the Illinois State Hospital for the Insane at Jacksonville, where she remained for three years. . . In a trial that received national publicity, Packard was declared sane. She then spent nearly two decades campaigning for the passage of personal liberty laws that would protect individuals and particularly married women from wrongful commitment to and retention in asylums (Grob 1994:84).

Packard focused on issues of rights protection and on abusive conditions of confinement. She found this combination of affronts to be particularly vile. She published several books, including *The Prisoner's Hidden Life, or Insane Asylums Unveiled* (1868) and *Modern Persecution, or Married Woman's Liabilities* (1874). She writes eloquently of the lack of rights protection for those who are confined: "Since there is no law to shield the insane person, he is, by law, subject to an absolute despotism. Thus the despot is protected in his despotism, no matter how severe and rigorous he may become . . . I cannot believe that there is any class of convicts or criminals in our land, who are not treated with more humanity—with more decency—with less of utter contempt and abuse, than you treat your insane patients here . . . Is there any spot in this great universe where human anguish is equal to what is experienced in Lunatic Asylums!" (Geller 1994:62-63)

Packard campaigned in several states for the passage of bills to protect people's rights not to be regarded as insane, and thus submitted to inhumane conditions, without proper evidence: "No person shall be regarded or treated as an Insane person . . . simply for the expression of opinions, no matter how absurd these opinions may appear to others" (Geller 1994:66), and "No person shall be imprisoned, and treated as an insane person, except for irregularities of conduct, such as indicate that the individual is so lost to reason, as to render him an unaccountable moral agent" (Geller 1994:67).

Packard's efforts resulted in legislative changes and influenced the work of Dorothea Dix, who started her own crusade for reform of state hospitals. Certainly Packard is an ex-patient who talked back to psychiatry. She is sometimes represented as a woman wrongly confined; other writers take pains to point out that she had been previously hospitalized (though it is not clear that casts doubt on her sanity).

Fifty years later, a man named Clifford Beers was calling attention to similar inhumane conditions in mental institutions. Beers' work is recognized as the inspiration for the "mental hygiene movement" which today is represented by the National Mental Health Association. He campaigned for recognition of mental illness as an illness that deserves humane treatment. In the preface to the 1981 edition of Beers' book *A Mind That Found Itself* (originally published in 1907), the Secretary of the American Association for Mental Hygiene states: "Clifford Beers must be counted as one of the mighty social reformers of the twentieth century. This book and a lifetime devoted to the development of community support for improved treatment and care, and for preventive services as well, have changed the course of our history" (Beers 1981:vii).

Beers had been confined for mental illness, then recovered and was released (though later re-hospitalized). He used his intellect, resources and personal connections, like Packard before him, to expose inhumane conditions and crusade for reform. Robert Coles describes Beers (in the Preface) as "a superb pamphleteer, propagandist, social and political activist—a man who knew how to negotiate those so-called corridors of power rather well" (Beers 1991:xiv).

The reformist advocacy position represented by Packard and Beers is both similar to and different from the c/s/x movement. Both speak with the actual voices of "ex-patients" rather than well-meaning but outsider advocates, to challenge inhumane conditions of treatment: "Is it not, then, an atrocious anomaly that the treatment often meted out to insane persons is the very treatment which would deprive some sane persons of their reason?" (Beers 1981:204)

Both call for legal reform to protect people from unjust incarceration, and promote the value of support, asylum and a sort of moral treatment under humane conditions for those who really require it. In that sense, they are calling for alternative treatment. Beers claims that: "Contact with sane people, if not too long postponed, means an almost immediate restoration to normality . . . it is the duty of those entrusted with their care to treat them with the utmost tenderness and consideration" (Beers 1981:204). He emphasizes that people do recover and need to be reintegrated into society without harmful stigma and stereotyping.

These two reformers fought courageously and publicly as socially, economically, and educationally privileged patients who had a glimpse of the madhouse, then obtained their release and called for reform. However, they did not organize their fellow sufferers, in fact they barely speak of them except as unfortunate victims and suffering souls. Instead, they organized sympathetic politicians and professionals in an effort to reform the abusive system they had both experienced, and to protect those inmates they had seen undergo such suffering. Beers worked to reduce the public stigma of mental illness, emphasizing that ex-patients do recover and must be allowed to enter the workforce and re-enter the normal world as productive citizens. He promoted the notion of prevention and early intervention as well as humane treatment, which led to the mental hygiene movement as mentioned above.

While Packard has received attention as a forebear of the Mad Liberation movement, unjustly incarcerated as an uppity wife with unusual behaviors (Chesler 1972; Szasz 1970), Beers is recognized as the originator of the mental health movement which resulted from "a national mass movement to prevent and to treat mental illness" (Beers 1981:vii). The Mental Health Association, which sponsors an annual conference named after Clifford Beers, is viewed by the more radical wing of the c/s/x movement as a more conservative, treatment-oriented group though it has recently been placing more emphasis on "consumer" concerns (this popularization and co-opting trend will be described below). For others, it represents an activist if conservative stance that focuses on education about mental illness and promotion of treatment.

An important point of contention is exemplified in Beers' statement that his doctors "had no difficulty in convincing me that a temporary curtailment of some privileges was for my own good. They all evinced a consistent desire to trust me. In return I trusted them" (1981:190). This phrase "for your own good" is a sort of derisive codeword in today's c/s/x movement that stands for the paternalistic and oppressive powers of psychiatry. In fact, it could be said that psychiatrists who truly desire to trust those in treatment might be those who are themselves supporters of the movement.

In effect, Beers represents a point of schism in the c/s/x movement, a schism that reveals the place between resisting and seeking treatment, between resistance and creating solutions that work in humane ways and do no harm. These early voices, precursors to today's movement, illuminate the conflicting yet continuous goals and themes of voice, rights and choice described above. In terms of the categories that emerged during the movement's history, Packard's position may be seen as a precursor to survivors/ex-patients, and Beers represents the precursor to the mental health consumer position.

## THE SEVENTIES: THE EARLY YEARS

### Speaking Out to Break the Silence

The era of the 1970s, with its social climate of rights awareness and social justice, and its challenges to expert authority, abuse of power and institutional control, marks the emergence of a larger movement for human rights in the mental health system. The early years of the movement are characterized by an increased awareness of the abuse of human rights in institutions, of the practice of psychiatry as social control, and of the inherent oppression of the psychiatric system to its workers as well as its patients/inmates. The growth of the movement included the exposure of abusive practices, the dissemination of dissident views in the field of mental health, and the promotion of rights protection for psychiatric patients, as well as the opportunity for development of a collective identity of dissenters from the mental health system.

### Dissenting Voices from the Mental Health System: Madness Network News

The early efforts to bring dissenters into the open and claim a voice are documented in the movement's first publication, the *Madness Network News (MNN)*. This newsletter began as a collaborative project by a group of disgruntled mental health workers and ex-patients in the San Francisco Bay

Area in August 1972 (Hirsch 1974), where radical activity in general was at a high level. Rights activism brought intense awareness of injustice and oppression, and a challenge to expert authority as well. The notion that mental patients were human beings with human rights was resonant with the public outcry about rights for women, blacks, homosexuals, the physically disabled, and other oppressed groups that were organizing for change.

The collaborative origins of *MNN* are worthy of note. From its beginnings, this collaboration represents the spirit of liberation and dissent shared by the early activists: psychiatric inmates, mental health workers, lawyers and psychiatrists, crossing the boundaries between providers and recipients of services. In fact, the funding source for the earliest issues of *MNN* was the SSEU (Social Service Employees Union). This radical dissident rag, which was distributed widely for free in psychiatric hospitals, clinics and on the street was funded by the workers' union; voices were raised by psychiatrized persons and workers together to protest the oppression of the mental health system.

The *MNN* started quietly, with a call for input and involvement from others who wanted to speak up about their experiences in the system:

> The newsletter is intended to be personal and informal. There is no editor [or] staff . . . just a group of friends doing it as it happens (although it's not just happening, we're making it happen—there wouldn't be a newsletter if we weren't). Anyone who wishes to contribute is asked to do so because that's what the whole thing is about and that is the only way it is going to continue to happen. We are particularly interested in printing the kinds of things everyone thinks about, but that very few really talk about, at least publicly, especially those things concerning the "knots"/Catch 22's/mind catch of the psychiatric system (*MNN* Vol.1:2, p.2).

This invitation prompted a powerful flow of information and narrative. The early issues of *MNN* exemplify the movement's spirit of inquiry, dissent and information-sharing. Expert knowledge about rights and treatment were exposed to public view, and experiential knowledge was claiming its own place at the table. The expression of previously unspoken subversive points of view had gained a platform and was coming out at rapid rate. Barriers between doctors and patients were broken down and dissenters were celebrated.

In each issue, the social concerns of the era are seen through the particular experiential lens of people in the psychiatric system. Major topics included patients' rights, protest against injustice and psychiatric oppression, involuntary hospitalization and forced drugging, alternative approaches to mental health, personal growth and creativity, and the meaning of madness. Writings by and about dissident psychiatrists (including Szasz, Breggin, and Laing) were focal points from the beginning as were articles about policies and laws relating to mental patient rights, about psychotropic drugs and their effects, and practices such as lobotomy and electroshock.

Dissident experts were showcased early on, and over time the voices and experience of ex-patients became more prominent. Here was mad liberation, a freedom movement on a par with women's liberation, gay liberation, and black power. Power to the people, and psychiatric patients are people too. The expressed goal of the *MNN* was to "Break the Silence": making private problems into public issues, exposing the abuses of psychiatry, educating people about the effects of psychiatric drugs, encouraging connections and dissent among those who had survived psychiatry and wanted to support each other both inside and outside the hospital.

### Spreading the Word: Building Collective Identity

As participation and response grew, the *MNN* actively promoted a growing sense of collectivity and identity formation among its readers: promoting a conference to bring people together, inviting reader input, seeing itself as just the beginning of a project in progress. Dissemination and monetary support were essential to spread the word. Subscriptions were requested from those who could afford them, and the goal was to publish monthly. By issue #5 in May 1973, there were "about 500 readers on our mailing list, two-thirds of them paid subscribers. We also distribute free about 1500 issues to psychiatric hospitals, both patients and staff, and some to organizations. . . Our readership includes so called 'mental patients,' therapists, administrators of hospitals, community mental health directors, artists, old people, ministers. We are primarily interested in the S.F. Bay area, but our readers extend nationwide and in Europe" (Vol. 1:5, p.2).

The solidarity across groups (dissident mental health workers and psychiatrists as well as patients and ex-patients) gave the newspaper a vitality of expression that was key to the growth of the movement, reflecting the inclusive radical approach to social justice that provided the context for its origins. Articles about oppressive working conditions and unequal power conditions for staff were reflected in the same light as oppressive conditions, psychiatric labeling, and harmful treatment for patients.

Psychiatrists wrote about their frustration as professional drug pushers and agents of social control, and shared insider expert information to empower those who might benefit. Lawyer-advocates wrote about promoting rights protection and new development in patients' rights law. Patients and ex-patients spoke out in their own words about abusive treatments, co-ercion, restraints, and incarceration. Published letters expressed support for the growing expression of voices that had been previously silenced, or heard only in secret. Dissident professionals joined with ex-patients to expose and transform the structures and practices of the mental health system. Some ex-amples of their voices follow in the next sections.

## Voices of Dissident Psychiatrists

The exchange of information was an important focus. "Dr. Caligari," a pseudonymous dissident psychiatrist, wrote informative columns about the dangerous side effects of psychiatric drugs. *MNN* members met with a group of mental health workers who "wanted to change the system but did-n't see themselves as capable of making changes and challenging the ac-cepted power of doctors . . . changing the system and make it truly respond to the needs of the people it pretends to serve" (1:6,7).

The radical psychiatrist Thomas Szasz, a hero of the movement from the origins to the present day, was featured regularly. Leonard Roy Frank described him this way:

> Thomas S. Szasz must present quite a dilemma to his colleagues in the field of psychiatry. After all, what do you do with one of your very own who regularly and openly blasphemes the gods of your group . . . he has denied the reality of mental illness and has de-nounced as criminals those who use the various classifications of mental illness as justifications for involuntary 'mental hospitaliza-tion' and coercive treatment (1:5,8).

Frank goes on to describe the relationship of Szasz to his profession in a way that presages the response of more conservative, authoritarian psychi-atry to the c/s/x movement itself: "Szasz's relationship with his profession is practically unique. He is like a barbed thorn in their flesh—if left in, it hurts: but the attempt to pull it out will cause greater pain, and what is more, may not be successful. So far his colleagues have largely ignored him, at least publicly. Authoritarians, whether political, religious or psychiatric, know that one of the most effective ways to repress heterodoxy is to avoid calling public attention to it . . . the tyrant's rule of no publicity for 'dan-gerous' ideas" (1:5,8).

A letter from a man in New Jersey described his plans to found a halfway house, based on his belief that "the attack on Institutional Psychiatry must be coupled with a struggle to affirm alternatives to hospi-talization for people in distress . . ." (1:6,10). This position represents the longstanding goal of the movement to provide alternatives as well as challenge psychiatric authority.

Other dissident psychiatrists and psychologists were included in *MNN* through articles, interviews, book reviews, compendiums of commentary on madness, etc. The voices of dissenting experts were a very important means to challenge and undermine the authority of the existing structures of the mental health system and encourage others to speak out against the dominant narratives of diagnosis and treatment. These voices would continue to be important allies through the next decades of the movement, though the focus would shift to the viewpoints and experiential expertise of those who had been objects of diagnosis and treatment.

### Voices of Ex-Patients: Finding Voice through Testimony and Witnessing

The voices of people who were psychiatrically labeled were an important feature of every issue of the *MNN*. These testimonies by present and former psychiatric patients represent a vitally important aspect of the movement and its history. The first year of *MNN* illustrates some of the earliest, at times tentative, efforts to speak out about the experience and "break the silence of psychiatric oppression." Over time, the voices of people labeled with mental illness would become even more central to the movement. Three examples:

"What It's Like to be Labeled Crazy" describes the experience of leaving the hospital to return to the community:

> My friends and neighbors looked at me and spoke to me strangely, and
> I felt like "a stranger in a strange land." Even my children had heard
> things whispered about me and didn't treat me normally. I thought that
> I would never make it back to society, and I found that I took the train
> from Connecticut into New York more and more often, so I could visit
> with friends I had made at the hospital, who seemed to be the only ones
> I could feel comfortable with, and were the only ones who "under-
> stood" me (1:5,5).

A page entitled "Shock" features the words of people who describe the horror, anger, and memory loss they and others had experienced as a result of involuntary shock treatments. One letter states, "I lost my treasured memory, and much of my mental ability. I used to be good at mathematics, now I'm just mediocre. I used to be the best bridge player at a hospital, now a retarded patient plays better . . ." (1:5,5).

On the same page, another ex-patient advertises a book entitled "The White Shirts" that describes her experience with 200 shock treatments and what she saw as the hypocrisy of the psychiatric profession (1:5,5).

*Finding Voice through Humor, Art and the Intellect*

The resistant identities of ex-patients and other oppressed groups were also expressed indirectly through alternative means—music, art, cartoons, and poetry. Contributions to *MNN* reflect this effort with a Mad Liberation theme. A "Festival of Creative Psychosis" sponsored by the Psychosis Validation Coalition featured "art, poetry and music done by mental patients and ex-patients" (1:5,11); a "Counter-Psychiatry" reading list was published with a request for more title suggestions (1:5,10). Art and poetry representing experiences with "madness" and the oppression of the mental health system is included in every issue of *MNN*.

A "Free University" course on Madness Inside and Out was described as follows: "Crazies, post-crazies, and pre-crazies from Madness Network News will lead a series of discussions on: Madness—Escape or Breakthrough?; The Place of Madness and Psychiatry in Current Social Change; Psychiatry and The Law; The Use and Misuse of Drugs; and Beyond Tyranny, Religious and Psychiatric. . . The staff of Madness Network News includes ex-inmates, a lawyer, a half-way house director, a psychiatrist a technician, a psychologist and various other folk" (1:6, 2).

A column by Leonard Frank heralded the development of specific movement humor directed back at those with the power to define. For example:

> CARDIOSCLEROSIS . . . hardening of the heart. Inability to feel sympathy for those who suffer. . . IN LOCO DEIS—a position of divine-like authority assumed by a psychiatrist in his relationship to the designated "crazy" person . . . PSYCHIATROPHILIA—love of psychiatrists. Affected persons accept without question all opinions and advice from psychiatrists who in reciprocation and gratitude regard them as the only truly sane members of society (1:6,9).

This "define the definers" humor has been ongoing throughout the life of the movement.

A woman in France reported on a meeting attended "by those who have been (or are) labeled 'crazies,' and stated, "I wrote to FOUCAULT (Michel)...and I sent him some photocopies of M.N.N. no. 4. . . He answered to me that he would write to M.N.N. Other French people must contact you" (1:6,10). Here we witness the growing international development of the movement, as well as its links to the intellectual contributions of Foucault, who had himself been quoted in a column on the definitions of madness in issue number four of the first volume.

And finally, a letter from the celebrated deviant and author Ken Kesey: "I'm into the first rewrite of the Cuckoo's Nest screenplay. But I haven't been in a nuthouse for more than ten years. Your paper came at a perfect time to remind me of something un-rememberable. Thanks . . . Long live Thomas S. Szasz!" (1:6,11)

## Voices of Lawyer-Advocates

Legal voices were also significant in *MNN*, and rights issues were reflected in community organizations. A task force on mental health for women was created at the California state conference of National Organization for Women (1:5,3); a conference called "Psychiatric Social Control—Bad Medicine!" was sponsored by the Citizens Commission on Human Rights in San Francisco (1:5,3). A new Center for the Study of Legal Authority and Mental Patient Status (LAMP) was highlighted with a regular feature about legal rights issues.

Growing concerns about civil liberties are illustrated by this quotation from a LAMP article about new court challenges to involuntary commitment procedures:

> Clearly, when a person is confined against his or her will, a civil liberties question is involved. The argument for "care and treatment" doesn't really hold water, because for most alleged "illness" the patient has a right to refuse treatment. Doctors have been saying that this right doesn't apply in commitment cases, because a "mental illness" is involved which only they, the doctors, are competent to diagnose and deal with. Now more people are beginning to understand that the inmates of mental institutions may be troubled, may be in pain, or may simply have been in the wrong place at the wrong time, without being "sick." In short, the "myth" of mental illness, as psychiatrist Thomas Szasz has called it, is under more critical examination. More people are coming to realize that the commitment process can be as much a power play as it is an exercise in "medical judgment" (1:6,4).

This excerpt refers to many of the core issues that would be paramount as the movement developed: coercion, the right to refuse, issues of power, social control and the medical model itself as applied to psychiatry.

## The First Conference

The first "Committee on Human Rights and Psychiatric Oppression" conference, held in Detroit in July 1973 was announced in the fifth issue. This conference showed evidence of national movement diffusion, with diversity of participants and topical issues:

for the first time ex-mental patients, consumers and professionals will join forces in an effort to bring about much needed change regarding the mental health system. The conference will have a workshop format to develop action programs to alleviate and eliminate problems. The areas to be covered at the workshops include the following: involuntary hospitalization; psycho-surgery, ECT, seclusion, behavior modification, and other "treatments"; patient advocate role of the professional; dehumanization; consumerism; legal issues; political action; legislation; drugs; long range planning of conference; community mental health; rights of minors; societal insanity; patients' rights; sexism (1:5,11).

According to Judi Chamberlin (1990), the conference was promoted by:

a sympathetic (non-patient) psychology professor and the New York City-based Mental Patients' Liberation Project (MPLP). Approximately fifty people from across the United States (and Canadian representatives) met for several days to discuss the developing philosophy and goals of mental patients' liberation. The leadership role of ex-patients was acknowledged; for example, the original name proposed by the sponsoring professor for the conference ("The Rights of the Mentally Disabled") was roundly rejected as stigmatizing (Chamberlin 1990:327 [81]).

After Detroit, conferences were held every year, providing a vital forum for networking and discussion as people came together from all around the U.S. to build the movement and support each other.

## Human Rights Issues

Another issue raised in *MNN,* and one that creates contention through the life of the movement, concerns fundamental threats to the human rights of the disempowered. These include, for example, a focus on research experimentation, sterilization, and the history of extermination of mental patients in Nazi Germany (Lapon 1986). A prominent article about The Committee Opposing Psychiatric Abuse of Prisoners is featured on the front page of the last issue of the first year of publication. The committee was raising concern about:

[the use of] human guinea pigs . . . [by] . . . the proposed Center for the Study and Reduction of Violence, being quietly implemented at the University of California. . . The center plans to utilize persons incarcerated in prisons and state mental hospitals as subjects of experimentation which will involve invasion of their mental and physical privacy. The use of these populations which are subject to coercion from state officials and do not possess many basic civil rights or the means of protecting them

raises serious questions about the meaning of "informed consent" in this
context. How can an individual under these constraints give voluntary
consent to being used as an experimental subject? Furthermore, the
Center will be focusing on populations primarily composed of black and
other Third World people (1:6,1).

These basic human rights issues have been a continuing theme and a light-
ning rod for conflict in the movement's history. People who are otherwise
sympathetic to the goals and themes of the movement are frequently of-
fended by c/s/x activists making reference to experimentation, Nazi extermination, sterilization, and other human rights violations. Such references
raise issues that benevolent normals, and well-behaved deviants, cannot always tolerate, and they provoke labeling responses like "paranoia" and extremism against the claims of the movement. Evidence is challenged and
accusations of exaggeration or poor judgment are brought into play. "Why
do they have to go too far like that, it just pushes people away and threatens their [our] credibility" (notes 7/16/02). Use of the term "survivors" of
psychiatry also pushes the limits of tolerance, which is not surprising when
even the term "consumer" feels threatening to the professional authority of
those who prefer the term "patient" (Torrey 1997; notes 9/29/00).

## Too Radical?

This righteous response to resistance and dissent, of social critique that
"goes too far," relates to Goffman's (1963) discussion of cranky or dis-
agreeable stigmatized persons who provocatively go beyond the "normals'" tolerance for being tolerant. "The stigmatized are fully expected to
be gentlemanly and not to press their luck; they should not test the limits
of the acceptance shown them, nor make it the basis for still further demands. Tolerance, of course, is usually part of a bargain" (Goffman
1963:120-121).

Accusations of "too radical" and "going too far" can come from inside and outside the movement, reflecting changing contexts and revealing
the (ultimately flexible) boundaries of the various factions and how they
choose to represent themselves to protect their own self-interests. For example, one activist, who edited what I considered a radical "zine," told me that
David Oaks of Support Coalition was "too radical for me" (personal conversation). On another occasion, at a meeting with a mixed group of mental health professionals and consumer/ survivors, an activist used the radical
term "inmate" when referring to patients at a local hospital. One of the professionals stopped the flow of talk to indicate that the use of such a term

was personally hurtful, offensive, inappropriate and divisive and should be avoided in the future (notes 6/22/02).

Over time, various interest groups made choices about where to stand on divisive issues. In the early years of the 1970s, however, these human rights concerns had continuity with other radical positioning about abuse of power. They were less of a threat, even an attraction, to the developing movement community.

## A Self-Aware Movement

The voices of dissident psychiatrists, ex-patients, and lawyer-advocates were creating momentum in *MNN* and the larger community. At the end of *MNN*'s first year of publication, the movement was in motion. In the fourth issue, the word "movement" was used with significant reflexivity: "Groups or individuals working within this movement may reprint articles but let us know first what you intend to use it for" (1:4,2).

That issue also featured a review of David L. Rosenhan's then-current study, "On Being Sane in Insane Places" (cited in *MNN* as being published that year in *Science,* Vol. 179, 1/17/73). The review described Rosenhan's now-classic critique of hospital staff's inability to distinguish pathology from normality as "another argument for the democratization of power throughout our society" (1:4,8). A Speaker's Bureau was announced, "available to speak to groups or organizations about many of the issues we discuss in the newsletter" (1:4,11). The movement was growing, with in-creased self-awareness of its burgeoning social movement status, but little sense of where it should be going.

The following reflective commentary in the fifth issue of *MNN* sum-marizes this situation:

> We started because we felt there was a big vacuum in the S.F. Bay area in regards to people labeled crazy along with the rights and dignity of "workers" and others in the psychiatric system or of anyone who might be touched by that system. At this point we feel we have done a lot to fill the vacuum, although there is still very little, if any, organizing hap-pening in the S.F. area regarding the issues that we raise. This summer we plan to take some time out from publishing the newsletter to get more involved in organizing, also to start working on a book . . . we will also be working on planning a conference to be held in the fall (1:5, 2).

The early goals of *MNN* were vague and open-ended, focusing on creating a platform for subjugated voices and the free expression of dissenting ideas. This unstructured approach kept the process open for growth and input from the community it was meant to reach. It was very successful in drawing upon the combined experiences of ex-patients and professionals to create a forum for speech and action. Without a hierarchy to create order and define goals (which would have destroyed its purpose), the emerging movement was shaped by the diverse concerns (and underlying power relations) of its participants. As it grew, the movement also faced an impending crisis of voice and power, to be revealed in the events that followed. The sources of this crisis of representation have continued to challenge the movement throughout its history, and indeed represent the challenge of its most fundamental goal: expressing the voice(s) of the psychiatrized. These historical factors are reflected in its evolving membership, factions and power struggles.

## Crisis of Representation

During the 1970s the momentum of the movement was building, and internal conflict developed between dissident professional voices and those of the psychiatrized. Although the presence of radical psychiatrists and staff had helped to galvanize the movement in the early days, as ex-patient voices grew stronger they found even such "benevolent" authority compromising to their deepest goals of finding authentic voice, representation, and self-determination.

In 1975, the third annual Conference on Human Rights and Psychiatric Oppression in San Francisco was the setting for a crisis of control. Judi Chamberlin described the situation in *MNN*. Whereas the two previous conferences had been designed with an open-agenda discussion-group atmosphere, this program "was transformed into a format in which 'resource people' presented topics, and 'facilitators' guided the ensuing discussions. . . The most glaring omission . . . was any discussion centered specifically around mental patients' liberation and mental patient organizing" (3:3,3).

Chamberlin continued with a description of the emotional state of the ensuing conflict, and what was perceived as

> the elitist professionalism that pervaded so much of the Conference . . . to de-emphasize and discredit the passion and anger of those Conference participants who live with the consequences of psychiatric oppression every day of our lives—former psychiatric inmates. Our individual expressions of anger and dissatisfaction were put down by some of the professionals present (supposedly our "allies") . . . areas of difference began to stand out clearly (3:3,3).

She then described a protest march at St. Mary's Hospital that happened the next day, in which former psychiatric inmates, who had been in a minority up to this point, were the clear and overwhelming majority of marchers. The anger that had begun to come into focus on Thursday grew stronger, as the realization dawned for more and more people that the professionals were far more eager to be leaders and teachers of mental patients than to confront an institution of psychiatric power (3:3,3).

Finally, Chamberlin describes how the experience of the protest march, after the angry disappointment of the previous day, became an important turning point for the movement:

The rally and march on Friday, July 4th was an exciting and unifying event. For the first time since the Conference began, we were a single force, united in confronting an outside enemy—St. Mary's "Hospital," both as an individual oppressive institution and as a symbol of the mental prisons nearly all of us had experienced. At noon, we gathered in Union Square in downtown San Francisco, where we listened to moving speeches by ex-patients from many parts of the country, and practiced the chants that would resound all along the lengthy march route. "What do you want? FREEDOM! When do you want it? NOW!" "Two, four, six, eight. Smash the therapeutic state" (3:3,4).

This powerful ex-patient movement energy was carried back to the conference, where:

a group of ex-patients called for a meeting, to be open to former psychiatric inmates only, to discuss formulation of a group response to the domination of the Conference by professionals and professionalism. It was at this point that we started referring to ourselves as the Ex-Inmates Caucus . . . for the rest of the Conference, most of the ex-patients could be found behind a door with a very clear "Keep Out" sign for anyone who hadn't done time in a mental institution (3:3,4).

The identity distinction had become clear. "It was truly as if there were two separate conferences going on—in one small, crowded, overheated room, we had recaptured the spirit of Detroit and Topeka [the two previous conferences]; while all around us, the hip shrinks, social workers, and others who claimed to be trying to 'help' us were holding their own dry, dull, deadly meetings" (3:3,4). And, in the final message of the conference: "The special status of ex-inmates within the anti-psychiatric movement means that professionals must be willing to challenge their own elitism and work with ex-patients *on our terms*. To appoint themselves the new experts is to maintain psychiatric power, not to combat it. If necessary, former mental patients can fight alone" (3:3,5).

The struggle for voice between ex-patients and dissident professionals continued. In 1976, after three years of publishing, the staff of *MNN* underwent a mutiny in which the non-patients were overthrown by the ex-patients, who took over the Madness Network collective. One of the departing staffers, Dr. David Richman, described the transition this way, emphasizing the difference between the earlier "broader movement" position and the recent "ex-inmate" emphasis:

> The original conception of the Madness Network was that it was not exclusively composed of ex-psychiatric inmates, but was a broader "coalition" of all those who shared common goals such as the abolishment of all forced "treatments" and forced psychiatric incarceration and Institutional psychiatry itself; and saw this as a part of a larger and broader movement to make basic changes in the nature of our world . . . one being the de-institutionalization of life. The gradual transformation of the Madness staff to totally ex-psychiatric inmates will be completed after this issue (4:1,2).

As the movement began to mature, and survivors/ex-patients built their own strengths through consciousness-raising and larger networks, they jettisoned the authority of what they regarded as well-meaning but oppressive experts. Chamberlin likens the process to other liberation movements:

> Among the major organizing principles of these movements were self-definition and self-determination. Black people felt that white people could not truly understand their experiences; women felt similarly about men; homosexuals similarly about heterosexuals. As these groups evolved, they moved from defining themselves to setting their own priorities. To mental patients who began to organize, these principles seemed equally valid [Chamberlin1990:325(79)].

As part of this process, the self-help philosophy of the c/s/x movement began to take shape. The core leadership of the movement in the 1970s were people like Chamberlin (1977), Howie the Harp (1984), Sally Zinman (1987), Leonard Roy Frank (1978), Su Budd, Jay Mahler (1997), David Oaks, Janet Foner, and Joseph Rogers, among others. All were psychiatric ex-patients with leadership roles in the movement, serving as inspiration to others as they shared the survivor stories that later became movement legends. Significantly, most continued as activists in the movement, and they are still active leaders, twenty-five and thirty years later.

All these individuals are white, though about evenly split by gender. This trend has continued at the levels of highest visibility, while at the local levels more racial and ethnic diversity is apparent. Some local leaders of color have become prominent at the national level as well.

The flexibility and ingenuity of the activists in finding each other, coming together, and building a movement is now the stuff of legend. Stories are told about their hospitalizations, their harrowing escapes from psychiatric confinement and abuse, then finding others who had similar experiences, sharing their anger, protesting abuse; also about the growth of the movement at annual conferences, held at campgrounds or college campuses, with just a few dozen dedicated activists who had hitchhiked across country to be there. The radical notion that former psychiatric inmates could help each other, without facing the harms of psychiatry, became a powerful force. Grassroots drop-in centers and self-help groups began to spread all over the country, with shoestring budgets or no budgets at all.

Self-help (later called peer support and mutual aid) became a rallying cry for the movement. Consciousness-raising groups were started all around the country. People who met in each other's kitchens, in church basements, or other safe spaces gradually became aware that there were many others who shared their experiences, their outrage, and their desire to make change. Other than the *MNN* and the annual conferences, there were no organizational structures motivating this movement. No national leadership or hierarchy was developed for several years, and that effort did not last long. This movement is not easily led. Self-determination is the key, and peer support provides the sustenance:

> At the same time that these mental health clients were struggling against the psychiatric system, they recognized that people did have emotional and other life problems and that they needed some place to go to for help and support (but without the coerciveness and oppressiveness of traditional mental health programs). Groups of psychiatric survivors, in the United States and in Canada, formed client-run alternatives to help meet their needs (Zinman et al., 1987:1).

It is important to note the emerging focus on combining advocacy with mutual support in the group meetings, as critical consciousness about psychiatry became more pronounced:

> While some were weekly support groups and other were centers and houses, most were also involved in advocacy. All these alternative groups were (and still are) meeting the needs of clients that were not met by the mental health system (in fact, the client's problems were often caused by the system—a situation which still exists today). For many years most

groups had little or no funding but, although they were relatively small, they produced impressive results. People in these groups had their needs met in very real ways and their lives were improved. For almost a decade, client-run groups helped hundreds of people, but remained virtually unrecognized by "the system" (Zinman et al, 1987:1).

## THE EIGHTIES: THE MIDDLE YEARS

### *Success and the Crisis of Co-optation*

Persistent demands for inclusion and voice, for representation in the mental health system and creation of alternatives, led to recognition and funding by bureaucrats at the national level. This development led to a further crisis, when centers gained funds and priorities were shaped by acceptability to funding streams. Survivor activism was partially co-opted by newly developing "consumer activism" and radical change agents saw their fellows transformed into mental health reformers.

Enmities and splits that developed in the face of success had repercussions for two decades, but the movement continued to grow and develop. Two streams could be identified into the mid-1980s, corresponding to those who sought funding and developed self-help groups, and the more radical faction that resisted co-optation. Self-help groups were embraced by the budget-conscious Republicans as a cost-effective way to use mental health funds, and the radical faction persisted in its activities and publication of the *MNN* until 1986 and then quieted, in a manner approaching abeyance (Taylor 1989).

Chamberlin described the changing era this way:

> I've never been sure where the term "consumer" came from, but I suspect it originated outside the growing community of activists, since its use seemed to coincide with the slowly growing recognition on the part of bureaucrats and service providers that they needed to develop mechanisms to listen to our message. At about the same time that we began to be invited to mental health conferences and the like, suddenly here was this new label that certainly was more comfortable for professionals than "mental patient," "survivor," or "inmate" (which were meant, in part, to be disquieting). Small amounts of money began to be available for the more acceptable, service provision end of our activities. Confrontational tactics like picketing and sit-ins became more and more rare (Chamberlin [1977] 2000:xii).

Gaining voice in provision of client-run services meant a loss of voice in the fight against forced treatment; but the fundamental themes of voice, choice, and rights continued to spread across the country at the grassroots level. The growth of seemingly innocuous drop-in centers for mental health "consumers" provided more safe spaces in which psychiatrized people spent time together, sharing their stories. Even centers that were closely supervised brought clients together in unstructured settings that espoused peer-run or peer-driven groups and self-help programming. Communication among centers increased as trainings and conferences provided a web of connections that were never possible before. The yearly conferences continued, and attendance grew.

## Claiming Voice at the Policy Level

Psychiatric patients and ex-patients found more seats at the table than ever before, as activists gained access to community mental health boards, spoke at hearings, and sat on committees. The process was not easy, as Chamberlin notes:

> Because most groups existed with little or no outside funding they were limited in their accomplishments. The question of funding generated numerous controversies, as did the question of reimbursement for organizational labor. Even if the group decided it had no objection in principle to receiving outside funding, obtaining such funding was difficult. . . Gradually, however, inroads were made. Members of ex-patient groups demanded involvement in the various forums from which they were excluded—conferences, legislative hearings, boards, committees and the like. Although at first in only the most token numbers, ex-patients were slowly invited to take part in such forums (Chamberlin 1990:329).

Gaining voice involves making demands, earning disapproval, fighting stigma and disregard, challenging the status quo. Chamberlin continues:

> Often groups had to insist on being invited, however. Once involved in such meetings, ex-patients could move in two different tactical directions: cooperation or confrontation. Clearly, much was said in these forums which directly contradicted the movement's developing ideology. . . Although ex-patients' objections to such mentalist assumptions were often used as a reason to exclude ex-patients from future meetings, it is to the movement's credit that the ex-patients did speak up and object to much of what was being said. Frequently-heard objections from professional participants were that the ex-patients "polarized the discussion" or were "disruptive." Professionals sometimes chose to work with non-movement-identified ex-patients who were much more likely to be compliant (Chamberlin 1990:329).

This shows the preference of the mental health bureaucrats for compliant "docile bodies" as representatives of consumer/survivor interests. Strident voices and demanding activists were a painful presence. Eventually, though, the efforts had the desired effect:

> The participation of ex-patients in CSP (Community Support Program) conferences . . . forced CSP to acknowledge the importance of funding patient-run programs as a part of community support. Such recommendations would not have been made—indeed, would not even have been considered—without the tenacity of movement activists who insisted on being heard (Chamberlin 1990:330).

Unfortunately, finding a seat at the table and gaining recognition from the mental health establishment resulted in a major schism in the movement. Disagreements over seeking and accepting federal mental health monies reflected the growth of a fundamental difference between "reform" and "rejection" of psychiatry as philosophical undercurrents in the movement. Reformers were seen by the radical wing as selling out, while the attraction of resources for creation of alternative programs was a powerful incentive to accept the funding, even if it meant fraternizing with the enemy.

### The End of Madness Network News (and of Anti-Psychiatry?)

*MNN* ceased publication in 1986. The last issue announced that the *MNN* collective was being dissolved. The co-optation of the movement with federal funds for community support and self-help programs, and increasing antagonism toward anti-psychiatry campaigns made this wing of the movement hard to maintain, as expressed in this farewell message: "Before we leave, we'd like to thank all of you who have been so supportive during the last several issues. This has been a very strenuous time for *MNN* and the anti-psychiatry movement. We, also, feel the strain. The effort by NIMH/CSP/APA to co-opt our movement with funding has been very successful" (*MNN* 8:3,2).

Two different endings to this column were printed (because the final draft was not approved before the collective dissolved). One ending was hopeful about continued resistance to psychiatric oppression; the second expressed frustration and doubt about the future, due to co-optation and distrust that had led to breakdowns of communication and movement solidarity:

> First Ending: Very few anti-psychiatry projects remain. But one thing is certain, no matter how unorganized the movement may currently appear the public-and underground-resistance to psychiatric assault and

psychiatric oppression will continue to grow. Psychiatry will one day be abolished. . . Second ending: A lack of real communication and trust in recent years among people has been another major cause of this success [in co-opting the movement] and continues to jeopardize what is left of our movement....Very few anti-psychiatry projects remain. Those that do tend to be isolated. It remains to be seen whether or not a visible, organized anti-psychiatry movement will continue to exist at this time (8:3,2).

This last issue of *MNN* demonstrates the dissolution of a movement institution (the Madness Network collective which had begun in 1972) which had provided a "centralized" focus for the growth of the c/s/x movement from the beginning. It appeared that the radical human rights and anti-psychiatry position most represented by the *MNN* was in peril. However, this same final issue in 1986 also provides evidence of an extensive network of local groups and individuals which maintained an ongoing life for the radical wing, in abeyance (Taylor 1989). The radical local groups continued to exist at the margins of the c/s/x movement during the next phase of growth, which would be characterized by the burgeoning self-help and mutual aid groups. Bitter competition, personal enmity and rancor characterized the split as the focus on psychiatric abuse and human rights issues lost ground and the movement gained power with emphasis on new areas described in the next section.

In this final issue we also have evidence of the powerful emotional energy and ideals of the anti-psychiatry position, in spite of its dwindling numbers and reduced influence. For example, a "Working Draft to Abolish Psychiatry" lists thirteen demands, beginning with "the immediate termination of involuntary psychiatric incarceration" and ending with "a just and humane society based on economic equality, mutual respect, and freedom." Similarly, a two-page photo spread features the "First Gathering of the Network to Abolish Psychiatry" held in Washington DC in May 1986 (8:3,8-9). An advertisement for the journal "Phoenix Rising: Voice of the Psychiatrized" (8:3,12) and news of "a resolution to abolish electroshock in Ontario" (8:3,10) provide evidence of continuing radical activities in Canada.

An indication of potential movement continuity is also present. A list of groups, with contact information, published in this last issue includes forty groups in the U.S., thirteen in Canada, five in the U.K., five in Holland, and seventeen more in seven other nations. Finally, a list of "those who want to form local anti-psychiatry groups" includes twenty-eight names and addresses (including David Oaks, soon to be editor of the *Dendron News,* which became the successor to *MNN* in 1988). Clearly, anti-psychiatry sentiments survived the death of *Madness Network News.*

*Consumer Self-Help: Empowerment and Co-optation*

The radical ex-patient stance was muted and moved to the background, while the reformist consumer position gained strength and recognition. The National Mental Health Consumers' Self-Help Clearinghouse, one of the major beneficiaries of the federally-funded "new era" of the movement, had been founded by Joseph Rogers, one of the figures in the contentious movement split over power and co-optation. As an example of the differing interpretation of the movement in the 1980s, this statement from his organization was much brighter than the message delivered by the last gasp of *MNN*.

First, this group stressed the reformist aspect of the new era:

> By 1980, individuals who considered themselves consumers of mental health services had begun to organize self-help/advocacy groups and peer-run services. While sharing some of the goals of the earlier movement groups, consumer groups did not seek to abolish the traditional mental health system, which they believed was necessary. Instead, they wanted to reform it. Consumer groups encouraged their members to learn as much as possible about the mental health system so that they could gain access to the best services and treatments available (National Mental Health Consumers' Self-Help Clearinghouse, n.d., 3).

Then, the empowerment aspect was stressed:

> Recipients of mental health services demanded control over their own treatment and began to have an influence on the public mental health system. Whether they considered themselves consumers or survivors, movement activists demanded a voice in mental health policy-making: a "seat at the table." Increasingly, they gained access to mental health policy-making and advisory committees. In addition, the number of peer-run services—drop-in centers, employment services, residences, and others—increased. Many of these services incorporated and received 501(c)3 (tax-exempt) status. Many received funding from federal, state, and local agencies. Studies found that peer-run services were effective, and cost-effective (NMHCSHC, n.d., p. 3).

In the second half of the 1980s, the self-help "consumer" movement became the face of c/s/x activism. The continuity of movement goals, with some changes, is evident: a focus on gaining voice, on access to knowledge and information, on choice, alternatives and self-determination. The emphasis, however, had moved to policy-making and program development. The earlier focus on rights and the challenge to psychiatry's powers of abuse and coercion was antagonistic to the mental health system and viewed as a threat to new "partnerships." Attention shifted to the challenge of obtaining funding, influence, and the power of negotiation, sitting at the table with professionals and policymakers.

Local groups continued to provide the heart of the movement in the mid to late 1980s. The self-help aspects of the movement were legitimized by federal funding and radical aspects were marginalized. Through the co-optation of the movement by federal monies (referred to in the final *MNN*, above), the annual conferences (still vital to movement activities) began to receive generous funding from the Center for Mental Health Services. This funding included scholarships that enabled many more individuals to attend. It also inevitably influenced the choice of topics and themes for the conference proceedings. What had begun as the "Annual Conferences on Human Rights and Psychiatric Oppression" became known as "Mental Health Alternatives" conferences. However these conferences, by providing an annual gathering place, continued to serve as the major organizing site for movement activities, and activists from all points on the radical-to-moderate continuum came to join together and participate in these meetings.

### Development of NAMI: "The Nation's Voice on Mental Illness"?

Another crucial development in the 1980s was the founding of the Alliance for the Mentally Ill, a support movement for the families of "the mentally ill" that advocated for more funding, better programs and improved psychiatric treatment for their family members. Sometimes derided as "NAMI mommies" by the c/s/x movement, the NAMI organization was able to develop enormous lobbying strength and greatly influenced NIMH funding for research on mental illness. E. Fuller Torrey (1988) describes their early lobbying efforts in his chapter entitled "Mothers March for Madness":

> . . . the families of persons with schizophrenia began coming out of the closets and organizing. Most of the family groups became affiliated as chapters of the National Alliance for the Mentally Ill (NAMI), and a rapidly growing advocacy movement was under way. By the mid-1980s NAMI groups had learned how to bring pressure on state and federal agencies. Some state mental health departments... began to reallocate resources to these patients. And the National Institute of Mental Health (NIMH)...began to talk of major new initiatives for research on schizophrenia (Torrey 1988:358-359).

Later in his "Mothers March" chapter, in a section on tactics for organized action, he encourages families to "lobby your Senators and Congressmen to put more pressure on the National Institute of Mental Health (NIMH) to shift research funds to schizophrenia and manic-depressive psychosis"

(Torrey 1988:372). (The first edition of his book was published in 1983.) Dr. Torrey also promotes making alliances with "patient groups" (and mentions the ideological changes in the c/s/x movement noted above): "Form an alliance with patient groups in your area to work on common interests. Patient groups are increasingly moving away from the rhetoric of Szasz ('schizophrenia does not exist') and Laing ('schizophrenia is a sane response to an insane world') and becoming effective in working for better services" (Torrey 1988:366).

Torrey promotes other strategies which have led to NAMI's remarkable effectiveness over the years: "Work to get representatives of family support groups on all city, county, and state mental health boards and advisory commissions, as well as the boards of directors of CMHCs (community mental health centers). . . Become expert on the county and state mental health budgets. Where is the money going? Who is getting services? Who is *not?*" (Torrey 1988:368).

Some NAMI goals and tactics can be seen to contrast with those of the c/s/x movement and would lead to future clashes over legal protections and mental health policy: "If laws in your state have tilted too far toward the patient's right to refuse treatment, begin a campaign to restore muscle to the laws, so that patients who need treatment will be treated. . . Advocate wider use of outpatient commitment laws, which permit patients to live in the community only so long as they continue to take medication" (Torrey 1988:371).

Finally, the next recommendation shows an ironic echo of the c/s/x movement, and also reveals the zeal of the NAMI membership for achieving its goals:

> Become the "lunatic fringe" of your local family support group. Threaten to lead marches of patients and families into county council meetings or state legislative meetings. Threaten to organize sit-ins at key offices or CMHCs unless specific needs of the seriously mentally ill are met. If necessary, carry out your threats. A "lunatic fringe" makes it easier for the mainstream majority in your organization to appear reasonable (Torrey 1988:373).

The current NAMI website states, "With more than 220,000 members, NAMI is the nation's largest organization dedicated to improving the lives of persons affected by serious mental illness." The group represents itself as "The Nation's Voice on Mental Illness" (http://www.nami.org). Not surprisingly, NAMI's growth in the 1980s and into the 1990s coincided with strengthened "brain disorder" models of mental illness as well as nationwide campaigns for more forced treatment. Although some c/s/x activists find solace in the "chemical imbalance" model and still work in advocacy for rights protection, NAMI's emphasis on "brain disorders" and promotion of forced community treatment programs are anathema to many in the c/s/x movement.

NAMI's fundamental claims to represent the interests of "the mentally ill" have challenged the voices of c/s/x activists from the start. After attending an early NAMI organizing conference, Chamberlin (1980) described the experience of encountering a group that claimed to represent "her voice" and advocate for "her interests" and her efforts to clarify the fact that "patients" were claiming their own voice:

> From the very beginning, there was a fundamental confusion between organizing parents' groups into a national organization, and promoting "advocacy" for the "mentally ill." These two purposes were stated interchangeably, and I felt that my main function at the conference was to make clear that it was impossible to speak of being the national advocacy organization without involving the ex-inmates' movement . . . Over and over again, in informal discussion and during meetings, I made the point that our movement would not stand silent and allow such a group to claim to represent patients. I emphasized that while our movement often disagreed with the positions of parents' groups, we would have no objection to their claiming to speak for parents, but the way they were proceeding guaranteed ex-inmates' opposition (*MNN* 1980,5:6,5).

The longstanding enmity between NAMI and the c/s/x movement is well-known in movement circles. It will be explored further in chapter five.

## THE NINETIES: THE RECENT YEARS

### Competing Ideologies and Interest Groups

The history of the 1970s and 1980s has been stressed in this chapter. These eras were important for the goal of gaining voice for the c/s/x movement. Through the process of gaining voice, along with access to knowledge and the power to define needs through self-determination, the movement began to develop different voices and competing ideologies. In addition, other advocacy voices like NAMI and various professional associations were also developing and promoting "consumer" interests in line with their own interests. By the mid-1990s, it had become quite trendy in the mental health system to invoke the "consumer" point of view. CMHS had hired a "Consumer Affairs Specialist" and NAMI had established a "Consumer Council." The National Association of State Mental Health Program

Directors (NASMHPD) gave extra weight to research that included a "consumer-researcher" or consumer presenter, and consumers were invited to attend their national research conferences for free (I was twice the beneficiary of this largesse).

These changes occurred primarily because more federal funds were designated to promote the incorporation of the consumer viewpoint into program development, research, evaluation techniques, and outcomes research. The consumer view was being recognized; it was also being commodified and homogenized, as well as pasteurized to cook out querulous contaminants. It was represented largely by selected members of the movement who had proven acceptable to the mental health establishment.

At the same time, the actual living variety of consumers, survivors and ex-patients were still at work in their local communities. Many were workers and participants at self-help client-run programs that had grown into a major segment of the mental health delivery system. Workplace settings involved partnerships with professional staff that, a decade prior, had been viewed as the enemy. Rights had been gained and protections were established. On the surface, the situation looked remarkably good.

But underneath the surface, the ongoing issues of voice and knowledge, rights, power and choice were still present. At the conferences, and behind the doors, c/s/x activists spoke about whose voices were being heard. With complacency in some areas, there was also a growing sense that movement successes had brought a loss of control over the terms of the discussion.

As the movement diversified, the 1990s also saw increased challenges to traditional c/s/x views on representation and voice at both local and national levels. In at least one state organization, strong minority leadership and representation, coupled with disagreements about whose views were being voiced, led to a threat of secession. Accommodations were made and the group did not split off. Though the psychiatrized master status often overrides differences of race, class, gender, ethnicity and sexual preferences, the process of coming to voice by identity groups within the movement has been ongoing, and may be tied to the growing maturity of the movement. Minority differences in experience of the mental health system, in experience of stigma, in personal or family response to emotional difficulties, and in power relations have brought the movement its own internal experience of identity politics.

### The Revolution of Internet Communication

The communication revolution of the Internet provided a resource for the self-help activities of the movement, zones of discussion for special interest groups, and a means to bring the radical wing back into action. At the systems level, some states created linkages among their community drop-in centers in order to coordinate mental health services while saving money on transportation and postage. Computer systems and technical assistance were provided in many settings. Extensive websites were developed for SAMHSA (Substance Abuse and Mental Health Services Administration), CMHS (Center for Mental Health Services), NMHA (National Mental Health Association), NAMI (National Alliance for the Mentally Ill), and the Self-Help Clearinghouse. Consumer Technical Assistance Centers (CTACs) received funding from CMHS to develop training and leadership modules to support and expand local self-help initiatives.

In addition, more radical individuals and groups developed elaborate websites with anti-psychiatry information, no-force discussion groups, alternative treatment programs, and news about recent developments in research and activism. Major sites include Support Coalition International, National Empowerment Center, MadNation, antipsychiatry.org, and many other advocacy sites in the U.S., Canada, and around the world (see Appendix B). Many of these sites have sponsored discussion groups to support connections among individuals around the country and the world.

With the Internet, information flows are instantaneous and access is enormous, ranging from MindFreedom and MadNation websites to those of the Journal of the American Medical Association and the Wall Street Journal. Activists are constantly monitoring the web for new developments from NAMI, the Treatment Advocacy Center, and other groups. Allies from other movements can communicate easily. Cross-national communication is instant and free. Thousands of people are accessing news bulletins, and campaigns or interventions can be put into action overnight.

## The Advent of Managed Care

In the 1990s, the strength of the movement began to challenge the mental health system in new ways. The advent of managed care programs changed the rules of the game, giving consumers-as-patients a bigger seat at the table in this market-driven model. Conference workshops were designed specifically to empower consumers to get the services they needed in the new era of managed care and medical necessity. Strategies were shared about how to maintain funding for drop-in centers and other "psychosocial" programming in a medically-based managed care environment.

Quality assurance and customer satisfaction became new vehicles for activists' voices. New entities called "consumer satisfaction teams" (CST's) were created to obtain feedback from consumers about their experience of mental health services. Mental health clients were being treated as customers who deserved to be satisfied; practitioners were expected to respond to their evaluation. Teams from around the country were able to join together for presentations at the annual Alternatives conferences, comparing notes on how to be successful and avoid being set up to fail by their mental health systems.

### Decade of the Brain and Radical Resurgence

The 1990s were declared by the U.S. Congress to be "The Decade of the Brain" (U.S. Dept. of Health and Human Services 1999:i). Ironically, this decade with its emphasis on biochemical and molecular solutions to human problems brought the radical movement back out of the closet. "The Surgeon General's Report on Mental Health" (U.S. DHHS, 1999) empha- sized the advances of research in understanding and treating mental illness, and encouraged people to seek help as they would for any other illness. A major theme of the report was the reduction of stigma attached to mental illness; another was the importance of treatment and intervention to reduce the "disease burden" (U.S. DHHS 1999:ix) of mental illness on the nation, including suicide. The Surgeon General's "Vision for the Future—Actions for Mental Health and the New Millennium" emphasized the ongoing need for scientific evidence-based treatment, for reducing stigma "by dispelling myths about mental illness," for providing accurate knowledge to ensure more informed consumers, and for encouraging help seeking by reducing barriers to treatment (U.S. DHHS 1999:xix-xx).

These recommendations may seem innocuous to the general reader. However, their goals of expansion of pharmacological treatment, stigma-re- duction through normalization of treatment, and parity of insurance care for mental illness (including forced treatment), and especially the potential for co- ercion toward treatment "adherence" brought a frenzy of objections from the c/s/x movement. The organized effort by NAMI and its sympathizers to intro- duce a PACT (Program for Assertive Community Treatment) model of forced outpatient treatment in every state mobilized a c/s/x activist force in the 1990s that was unprecedented in the history of the movement. Between NAMI and the new pharmacological psychiatry, the threat to freedoms and human rights in mental health once again became a top priority for the movement.

### Human Rights Resurgence

The international movement for human rights in psychiatry also gained ground in the 1990s. Activist organizations all over the world joined Support Coalition International, bringing the number of member groups to one hundred. More participants from Canada and Europe attended the annual conferences, and the conversation has grown. The radical position on human rights in psychiatry has been maintained since the 1970s, seemingly in abeyance (Taylor 1989) as the more conservative factions were more visible in their more socially-acceptable resistant roles.

Yet the radical activists were networking in the background and these activities led to recent gains. The radical Support Coalition International (SCI) group developed strong alliances in the global human rights movement and achieved consulting NGO status in the United Nations. Nine members of Support Coalition International obtained credentials to attend the UN Ad Hoc meetings on disability and human rights, and SCI achieved Non-Governmental Organization Consultative Roster Status with the UN's agency ECOSOC (SCI email 7/26/02). This recognition adds legitimacy and influence.

### Public Exposure for Dissenting Voices

The c/s/x movement has worked to alert the public to the dangers of psychiatric drugs and electroconvulsive treatment (ECT), with some success. A muckraking article about the pharmaceutical money behind NAMI's organization was published in *Mother Jones* (Silverstein 1999). The popular press published such challenges to traditional psychiatric practice as *Your Drug May be Your Problem* (Breggin and Cohen 1999) in which safe withdrawal from psychiatric drugs is explored, and Dr. Loren Mosher's article "Are Psychiatrists Betraying Their Patients?" in *Psychology Today* (Mosher 1999) which described his resignation from the American Psychiatric Association to protest the power of pharmaceutical companies in psychiatric practice: "Why does the world of psychiatry find me so threatening? Because drug companies pour millions of dollars into the pockets of psychiatrists around the country, making them reluctant to recognize that drugs may not always be in the best interest of their patients" (Mosher 1999:41).

## 2000 AND BEYOND: THE EMERGING YEARS

The increasingly radical activities of the movement continued into the new millennium. Support Coalition held two strategy conferences in 2000 and 2001, at Highlander Center in Tennessee, the legendary site of celebrated social movement activism. This meeting brought thirty leading activists together to develop strategies for the next phase of the movement. A "Highlander Statement and Call to Action" was produced at the 2000 meeting. This call for action was posted on the SCI website and distributed widely after the meeting. Following are excerpts from the statement:

> We call upon all people committed to human rights to organize and
> fight against the passage and implementation of legislation making it
> easier to lock up, shock, and forcibly drug people with psychiatric dis-
> orders . . . to work together to build a mental health system that is based
> upon the principles of self-determination . . . to heal each other by
> telling our stories . . . we call upon elected officials, political candidates,
> and those with power over our lives to recognize and honor the legiti-
> macy of our concerns (Highlander Statement, March 25, 2000).

Several SCI members followed up the conference by arranging a visit with
the staff of Vice-President Al Gore to discuss mental health policy issues.
The timing of the 2001 meeting coincided with a campaign against forced
ECT in New York (see chapter five); the organizing efforts were energized
by strategies developed at the conference to be put into action by participants at the hospital site. The mystique of meeting at Highlander provided
an identity boost for the movement, with a new sense of legitimization and
power that included new recruitment strategies, especially of youth and minority members, and renewed efforts to expand coalitions with other rights
groups. The library at Highlander now includes books about the c/s/x
movement on its shelves, donated by Support Coalition Strategy
Conference participants, and the activists were energized by the planning
meetings in the Smoky Mountains. The third annual SCI Strategy
Conference in 2003 was moved to another site in Kansas in response to
members' needs for more accessible facilities.

### Growing Influence of the Movement

Since 2000, the movement's influence had grown in the media and at policy
levels. There was more attention in the mainstream press, reflecting a larger
presence in the circles of mental health policy-making and practice. Two
new books that critiqued psychiatry and included information on the c/s/x
movement were recently published: *Mad in America* by Robert Whitaker
(2002a) and Bruce Levine's *Commonsense Rebellion* (2001). These books,
reviewed in the national press, appeared on the shelves in public libraries
along with new works by Thomas Szasz entitled *Pharmacracy* (2001) and
*Liberation by Oppression* (2002). Movement ideas were increasingly available in the mainstream.

Ron Bassman, Ph.D., a psychologist and movement leader who was
once diagnosed with schizophrenia, published an article in *Psychology
Today* (Bassman 2001) that described the story of his horrific incarceration and treatment. Ron told me he had mixed feelings about the article:
he felt that he was exploiting his story, but wanted to get the word out. He

explained the concept and experience of recovery in the article, first describing his encounters with psychiatry:

> When I was discharged from the hospital I was told I had an incurable disease called schizophrenia. The doctor told my family that my chances of being re-hospitalized were very high. His medical orders were directed at my parents, not me, and stated with an absolute authority that discouraged any challenge. He predicted a lifetime in the back ward of a state hospital if his orders were not followed. . . The hospital doctor put me into a coma five days a week for eight weeks by injecting me with insulin. Those 40 insulin treatments combined with electroshock blasted huge holes in my memory, parts of which have never returned (Bassman 2001:36).

He went on to describe the term "psychiatric survivor" which is not often heard by the general public, and the "closeting" of people who successfully recover yet prefer to avoid the stigma of their current or former psychiatrization. Bassman's own voluntary "outing" of himself as a successful psychiatric survivor brought a voice from the movement into a mainstream popular magazine:

> My best friends were once locked up in mental hospitals and fought their way back. We are psychiatric survivors. Some believe that psychiatric survivors defy the odds. Or maybe we were never really mentally ill, just misdiagnosed. After all, they say schizophrenia is a lifelong disease. Such reasoning makes my peers and me look like exceptions. Among our large group of closeted ex-patients are lawyers, teachers, mechanics, doctors, carpenters, plumbers and psychologists. We are your neighbors, ministers and friends, living and working in your communities. Many thousands choose not to reveal their past. I choose to speak and write about my experiences so that others who have been diagnosed and treated for serious mental illness will be able to see new hope and possibility (Bassman 2001:36).

Similarly, Joseph Rogers, a movement leader of the National Mental Health Consumers' Self-Help Clearinghouse, was featured in *U.S. News & World Report* in June 2002. Meanwhile, his center's funding was endangered by the threat of federal cuts to Consumer Technical Assistance Centers. This news magazine provides a well-informed view of both Rogers and the consumer movement:

> For the past 18 of his 50 years, [Rogers] has been one of the leaders of the mental health "consumer movement." Since 1997 he has been executive director of the Mental Health Association of Southeastern

Pennsylvania, a $12.1 million organization that runs 30 programs for the mentally ill in Philadelphia and surrounding communities. Most of its 326 employees are, like Rogers, consumers (their preferred label, which they consider less stigmatizing than the many others). Says Estelle Richman, Philadelphia's health commissioner: "Without Joe, our system would not be what it is today. It would not be nearly as responsive to the needs of consumers . . ." (Szagedy-Maszak 2002:55).

The article goes on to describe more about the movement's goals and history:

Rogers is one of thousands of people suffering from brain disorders who have radically changed how services are delivered to the mentally ill. Their mission is simply stated: to encourage self-help, eliminate stigma, emphasize recovery, and provide hope to those with mental illness. The movement is a curious hybrid of the 1960s civil rights movement and more-recent health advocacy efforts—for AIDS and breast cancer, for example (Szagedy-Maszak 2002:55).

It is characterized as a "mainstream movement" with a part in the policy process:

Although it began with a marginalized collection of former mental institution patients demanding the closure of state hospitals, today it's a national, mainstream movement, representing the entire array of psychiatric diagnoses and challenging psychiatrists and other "helping professionals." The first surgeon general's report on mental health, issued in December 1999, stated: "Consumers are now seen as critical stakeholders and valued resources in the policy process" (Szagedy-Maszak 2002:55).

Clearly, there is a new visibility of c/s/x activists in the mainstream press, reflecting their presence in the circles of mental health policy-making and practice. The movement is having an effect, and its voices are being heard. Indeed, such characterizations in the media are strong evidence that the movement has already had a significant effect, and will continue to do so. Yet the different representations create a new arena for conflict.

The film *A Beautiful Mind* provided an opportunity for debate about the use of psychiatric drugs. In the film, John Nash resumed taking his medications and obtained recovery from his hallucinations, later winning the Nobel Prize. In real life, and in the biography by Sylvia Nasar (1998), Nash quit taking his medications in 1970 and never started again. To quote Nasar:

Nash's refusal to take the antipsychotic drugs after 1970, and indeed during most of the periods when he wasn't in the hospital during the 1960s, may have been fortunate. Taken regularly, such drugs, in a high percentage of cases, produce horrible, persistent symptoms like tardive dyskinesia—stiffening of head and neck muscles and involuntary movements, including of the tongue—and a mental fog, all of which would have made his gentle reentry into the world of mathematics a near impossibility (Nasar 1998:353).

Nash became a hero to the c/s/x movement, and the medication controversy provided an opportunity to speak out. A Support Coalition news release by David Oaks (3/6/02) refers to a *USA Today* article by Robert Whitaker and states:

> The film is helping millions admire the resilience of psychiatric survivors. But this film also seriously misleads the public. The fact is, many people—like Nash—recover without taking psychiatric drugs. By caving in to pressure, the film has become an advertisement for the psychiatric drug industry. Nash himself wonders if the fact that one of the film's writers is related to a psychiatric professional played a role in this distortion (SCI news release 3/6/02).

Whitaker's *USA Today* commentary further notes: "In the movie, Nash—just before he receives a Nobel Prize—speaks of taking 'newer medications.' The National Alliance for the Mentally Ill has praised the film's director, Ron Howard, for showing the 'vital role of medication' in Nash's recovery. But . . . this brilliant mathematician stopped taking anti-psychotic drugs in 1970 and slowly recovered over two decades" (Whitaker 2002b:13A).

Another commentator in the SCI news release, Barry Duncan, PhD notes that Nash's story "predates the so-called 'newer psychotics' by some 20 plus years" and wonders, "does drug company marketing now include product placement in the movies?" (SCI news release 3/6/02) Such opportunities for debate may have some impact on the public view of the issues. They also provide an opportunity for the voices of c/s/x activists to speak to each other and respond to media issues, to work with the play of power in the expression of points of view, and to build solidarity with movement allies.

### A Countermovement Backlash

The backlash against the movement has come most strongly from those that David Oaks labels "extremist psychiatrists" who are working to maintain their control over people labeled with psychiatric diagnoses—especially people who talk back, who deny they need treatment, or choose to decide what treatments they will accept. These psychiatrists have the ability to influence policy and funding. Chapter five includes a discussion of the campaigns and counter-campaigns, as "extremist psychiatry" responds to movement success with efforts to destroy its credibility and federal funding.

### Success Brings More Risks

Clearly, evidence from the 2000s shows that the movement has had an effect. Movement influence has entered the mainstream in both its moderate and radical forms. These news stories, these cash flows, these influential positions, would never have been dreamed of in the 1970s. Yet there are big risks, as the loss of funding could be devastating. The old arguments about taking money and co-optation start to ring true as the Bush Administration threatens cuts to the longstanding federally-funded consumer self-help initiatives. Funding for all forms of mental health programs faces cuts as states struggle with huge deficits. Support for consumer programs, developed in the Reagan administration and well-established since then, is being withdrawn with encouragement from psychiatrists who want to reassert their expertise and emphasize the power of biomedical and psychopharmacological interventions.

For the more radical activists who have never taken government or drug money, this "defunding" moment has been a bittersweet moral victory. Yet, ironically, the two sides of the movement came together in the face of this crisis, as the significant funding and credibility gains of the past two decades were threatened. Two strong-willed individuals, David Oaks and Joseph Rogers, both long-time movement leaders who shared enmity and disdain for many years as the movement split, found ways to cooperate, however reluctantly, to keep the movement alive. They each rallied their own supporters, joining forces with the physical disability movement after the death of another movement leader, Justin Dart on June 22, 2002. With the inspiration of Dart's final call for solidarity, justice and empowerment (SCI e-mail 6/22/02), they and other movement members joined in a concerted effort to maintain the gains of the past two decades and fight the power of conservative policymakers and the pharmaceutical industry. There was too much to lose. This was a significant shift in movement strategies; its results remain to be seen.

### Meeting the Challenge

These are the forces that characterize the emergence of the c/s/x movement into the new century. Given its history it is likely that this movement, whatever the challenges, will persevere in some form as it has for thirty years: gaining voice, providing choice, fighting for rights, and telling truth to power. In September 2002, David Oaks of Support Coalition delivered the keynote speech at the Alternatives Conference in Atlanta, Georgia. The excerpt included here demonstrates the new themes of a movement that will overcome historical differences and include diverse points of view. The undercurrent of longstanding difference and resolution are evident as he emphasizes the effort to make a "big enough" movement for everyone:

> Our movement can be big enough for choice and different points of view. When one person says psychiatric drugs saved my life and helped me recover, and another person answers, psychiatric drugs poisoned me, I'm now drug free and fully recovered, that is not necessarily an argument. It is the sign of a strong movement. Our movement is big enough for people who currently use the traditional psychiatric system, and our movement is big enough for people like John Nash, the hero in the film A Beautiful Mind, who actually quit all psychiatric drugs back in 1970. Our movement is big enough to use inclusive language such as mental health consumers and psychiatric survivors. We are all united for freedom of the mind. . . Our movement is big enough to include both government funded groups, and independently-funded groups. In fact, our whole movement needs to raise more funds with no strings attached. . .

and a call for unity, activism and shared commitment to justice:

> Our movement can be big enough to link the two engines of our movement. We can link the powerful gears of mutual support, with the mighty gears of activism. . .Our movement is being challenged as never before. But we must remember our people have survived so much. Many of you here—if you want to call out—have like me survived forced psychiatric drugging. You survived the isolation of solitary confinement. Some of you survived electroshock. You survived the despair of homelessness. You survived poverty. You survived restraints. You survived discrimination. And yet you have not been stopped. We will not be stopped. Nothing can stop the power of love and the struggle for justice" (http://www.mindfreedom.org/mindfreedom/conference.shtml).

The consumer/survivor/ex-patient movement has shown evidence of growth and strength in the face of adversity and threat. If members and leaders are able to overcome their differences and work together effectively, especially in alliance with other justice movements, they may continue to gain a stronger voice. Their adversaries are formidable, influential and well-funded; yet the fight against forced treatment and psychiatric oppression has not stopped. True to its origins, the c/s/x movement continues to emphasize the importance of gaining and maintaining voice, promoting and protecting rights, developing alternatives for choice, and exposing the knowledge claims and practices of psychiatry. "Breaking the Silence" and "Ending Psychiatric Oppression" are ongoing endeavors.

Chapter Four
# Resistant Identities: Voice, Choice, and Advocacy

> The struggle to end domination, the individual struggle to resist colonization, to move from object to subject, is expressed in the effort to establish the liberatory voice—that way of speaking that is no longer determined by one's status as object—as oppressed being. That way of speaking is characterized by opposition, by resistance. It demands that paradigms shift—that we learn to talk—to listen—to hear in a new way.
>
> —bell hooks (1989:15)

## INTRODUCTION

The previous chapter explored the two intertwined themes that give an identity to the c/s/x movement. The themes of Breaking the Silence and Ending Psychiatric Oppression reveal the important movement goals of claiming voice, gaining access to knowledge, claiming and protecting rights, challenging oppressive authority, exposing abuse, and creating choice by developing opportunities for alternatives and self-determination. We have seen how the continuity and change of the movement over its history reflect an interaction of these themes with the social, economic and political contexts of the times. In this chapter, the interplay of these themes in individual resistant identities will be explored.

Data for this analysis derive mainly from the in-depth interviews, conversations and presentations heard through participant-observation, and personal stories obtained through archival research; all are rich sources of narrative describing the path into psychiatric treatment and then into activism. Participants at various levels of involvement in the movement eloquently describe this process of identity development. Similar themes appear in the narratives of local advocates and national leaders, recent arrivals and radical long-term activists.

This chapter explores the experiences and interpretations that illustrate people's resistance of the "mental patient" identity in relation to psychiatry, and the experiences that motivate them further to advocacy, both self-advocacy and advocacy for others. In small and large ways they talk back and resist the influence of psychiatric power in determining their lives, and help others to do so. The goals and values of the c/s/x movement become defining factors of identity for these advocates, and help to shape their experience of treatment in the mental health system. At the same time, these experiences help to reinforce the goals and values of the movement. The larger movement is built on the experiences of people at the grassroots level, and their power is reinforced by the energy and support of the movement.

Recognition, activation, and reinforcement of the movement's themes and goals by psychiatrized individuals are fundamental in defining its membership. Development, maintenance, sharing, and celebration of "resistant identities" are core features of the c/s/x movement and an important part of the conferences and publications. Awareness of shared experiences and interpretations becomes the basis for consciousness-raising that leads to a sense of collective identity and being a part of something larger.

Committed members of the c/s/x movement express an awareness of the injustice of psychiatric oppression, a willingness to speak out, and the desire to work for change in pursuit of the movement goals delineated above. Anger and betrayal are underlying emotions expressed by many at the conferences. "Never again" is a theme of activism that is continuous as members describe involuntary treatment and confinement, being subjected to four-point restraints, seclusion rooms, and demeaning and abusive behavior by professional staff "in the name of help."

To avoid having similar experiences again and again as they are hospitalized and lose their power of choice, some movement advocates promote the use of legal documents called advance directives, designed specifically for psychiatric treatment. These are documents in which the individual, who is certified to be competent at the time, makes clear statements about preferences regarding treatment conditions to be preferred or avoided when they are next hospitalized. In New York State, a group called The Alliance created a registry for advance directives, making them available in a centralized place to be consulted whenever a person was hospitalized. These documents are a way to encourage the "collaborative approach to chronic illness" described in chapter one. If they are taken seriously, psychiatric advance directives (PAD's) are a way for people to have input into the choices made for their treatment—what works, what is harmful, what doctor or hospital or medication has been helpful or harmful to you in the past?

Some strong supporters of the movement have not themselves been psychiatrized yet they have been exposed to betrayal or injustice in the mental health system, whether personally or through their work or their relationships. Legal advocates, psychiatrists, and other mental health workers, as well as some family members who do not agree with the NAMI views, have formed dynamic and longstanding alliances with the movement. These allies demonstrate remarkable depth of commitment to c/s/x values and goals, even when their alliance has caused them to be ridiculed or rejected by their own "normal" peers and professional colleagues.

I will use the framework of "heroic survivor narratives" of the larger movement, along with examples from my interview data, to present an analysis of the forms of resistance to psychiatry revealed by movement activists. Their resistance is expressed through interpretation of their experience, their sense of discrediting or injustice, and their choices of how to respond through speech, action, and advocacy. Not everyone is a heroic survivor; not everyone is an activated consumer. The similarities and differences reveal an underlying structure that enlarges the understanding of resistance, the experiences of psychiatrization, and motivations for action among members of the movement.

## HEROIC SURVIVOR NARRATIVE

The celebration of resistant identities in the c/s/x movement is personified by a collection of heroic survivor narratives. Chamberlin's *On Our Own* (1978) Kate Millett's *The Loony-Bin Trip* (1990), Shimrat's *Call Me Crazy* (1997), and Wendy Funk's *What Difference Does it Make (The Journey of a Soul Survivor)* (1998) are important examples of heroic accounts by individuals who survived the challenge of their encounters with psychiatry. *Shrink Resistant* (Burstow and Weitz 1988), *Beyond Bedlam* (Grobe 1995), *Cry of the Invisible* (Susko 1991), and *Madness, Heresy and the Rumor of Angels* (Farber 1993) are examples of edited collections of personal accounts. Personal narratives of surviving, outwitting, or avoiding psychiatry appear regularly in movement publications and provide an important segment of programming at annual conferences.

These narratives play an important part in the movement's development and maintenance of collective identity. The experience of membership builds on the resonance of these stories with individual experience, and it is reinforced through the repetition of personal accounts. Narratives of survival are a tradition and a recruitment tool for the movement. They provide a means to frame one's own experience with psychiatry, to experience a collective recognition or shared injustice, and to identify with the power of heroic accounts.

Leonard Roy Frank's story is told in Farber's (1993) collection, and Sally Zinman's in *Madness Network News* (also recounted during an Alternatives 1999 plenary session). I will not do justice to their experience by summarizing in this way, but simply expose the structure of the stories. Both were put into treatment after their behaviors became incomprehensible to their concerned parents: Leonard grew a beard, became vegetarian, and spent all his time with books; Sally stopped wearing makeup and expressed alienation from her parents. She also stopped using her name.

Their stories describe the betrayal funnel (Goffman 1961) experience noted earlier, as both entered treatment they then found to be extreme and abusive: Leonard received insulin shock and electroshock treatments from his doctors and Sally was locked in a cellar and abused by hers. Both attempted to escape, first by reasoning with their captors and then by resisting (Sally ran away and was forcibly returned with the help of her parents; Leonard refused treatment and was treated against his will); both were discredited, punished and received further treatment, as their efforts to resist and talk back were interpreted as signs of their illness.

Over time, both realized that their best strategy was to be convincingly "normal" and stop arguing or fighting back. Convincing the treatment professionals that their treatment had worked became the best way to gain their freedom. Both described the "never again" determination to prevent this from happening to others if they survived. After release, they discovered other people who had survived similar suffering and joined with them in activist alliances to protect rights of patients and expose psychiatric abuse. Leonard was an early member of the *MNN* collective and has been active in the movement since its earliest years; Sally has been active since the 1980s and continues to be a leader of the California Network of Mental Health Clients. Similar accounts appear in the other examples listed above.

These heroic survivor narratives reveal a five-phase framework of experience that is quite consistent across examples. The structure provides a model for understanding the process of identity transformation in the creation of resistant identities. Not everyone goes through all these phases in orderly or linear fashion, and they are not meant to provide an "evolutionary" model of experience. Rather, they serve as examples of forms of resistance in relation to treatment, to professionals, and to other psychiatrized people. I will describe the framework of survivor narratives in the next section, and then compare "ordinary" grassroots activists' experiences of psychiatry (my interview data) to the heroic framework presented. This comparison reveals the range of responses that characterize "resistant identities" in relation to psychiatry and aids in understanding the complexity of movement membership and experience.

## PHASES OF HEROIC SURVIVOR NARRATIVE

### *Entry into System: Trust/Distrust*

Some activists describe an initial recognition of the need to seek help for distress or disturbance, and a voluntary entry into the patient role. Others describe an involuntary introduction to this process. They often make a good-faith effort to benefit from help, because they have hope, or because they have no choice. They may initially believe in the doctor's authority and in put their trust in the psychiatric diagnosis, complying with their designated treatment. Later, they perceive that the treatment is not helping, or is causing them harm. In an alternate form, they may not have the initial period of trust and describe only their experience of harm and abuse. Through whichever route, each individual comes to the point of finding the "help" to be harmful.

### *System Disregard: Discrediting Personal Realities*

Survivor narratives go on to describe the experience of harm being compounded by a disregard for their efforts to define the experience, to negotiate the terms of treatment, or to leave the situation. Their sense of betrayal (if trust was achieved) and their disappointment that their own experiential knowledge of the situation can be so discredited is a powerful aspect of the accounts. The heroic narrative describes the transformation from ordinary human being to mental patient, with the realization that the psychiatric label destroys the credibility one may still expect to have in human interaction.

### *Resistant Response: Refusing Incorporation*

In this pivotal phase of the survivor narrative, efforts to negotiate on the basis of trust and reason are abandoned. The master status of mental patient identity and its discrediting consequences are rejected, with an effort to maintain a positive identity of the self. These activists resist the internalization of deviant identity, and the resultant incorporation of (into) the psychiatric narrative. After varying lengths of time, some form of personal heroism or assistance from others will result in a personal victory involving symbolic and/or physical escape from psychiatric oppression.

## SOLIDARITY: RECOGNIZING SHARED OPPRESSION

Activists may frame their heroic narratives as individual experiences of survival, with a later recognition of shared oppression and a wish to prevent it from happening to others. In other cases, an experience of shared awareness serves as the source of recognition of oppression. In either case, the experience of solidarity is a vital part of the movement's survivor narratives. Individual survival is not enough; some form of consciousness-raising leads them to an experience of collective identity.

### *Politicization: Making Demands for System Change*

In this phase, activists move beyond their experience of shared oppression to an activist position. With their peers, they develop a motivation for challenging the status quo by exposing the situation of oppression and abuse. They move beyond personal experience and take a politicized stance, recognizing their shared experience as a reason and a catalyst for creating change. Then they take action based on their views of injustice, available methods to gain and use power, and objectives for change.

   The survivor discourse of this movement shows similarities and differences when compared to discourses of incest and rape survivors (Naples, 2003). The struggle for voice is central, and the goal of finding credibility (to self and others) while legitimizing one's experience, including the identification of a perpetrator, are vital parts of the process. There are also similarities in the struggle for control over the discourse between psychiatrists and consumer/survivors and a critical praxis is important. In the case of c/s/x survivors, consciousness-raising is central because the perpetrator has been the provider of help, and the move away from a therapeutic relationship toward peer support is often the focus of the narrative. There are many interesting questions about the relationships of power, discourse and identity in these contrasting survivor experiences that can profit from deeper examination, though they will not be explored here.

## LINKING INTERVIEW DATA TO HEROIC SURVIVAL NARRATIVE

I was familiar with the heroic movement narrative (Chamberlin 1978; Farber 1993) when I began my research. This exposure had probably framed my expectations of movement activists and my views of what a "resistant identity" might entail. In the process of fieldwork and collecting the interview data, I met more local-level or ordinary activists, and became aware of the range of experiences that counted as movement activism. Through talking with many activists in the field, and collecting the interview data, I learned that resistance comes in many forms. Resistant identities incorporate these different forms and become the people who constitute the movement.

Recognition of these various forms of identity has led to a greater understanding of the c/s/x movement as a whole, with its internal tensions and challenges and the diversity of its members. An individual may reject psychiatry or take medications, may have been hospitalized or not, may have experienced severe abuse, or may have avoided it. These factors help to shape the forms of the multiple movement identities; the consumer/survivor/ex-patient (c/s/x) differences are enacted through individual experience and interpretations. Yet this full range of experience is included in the movement, and people who personify the different aspects identify themselves as members of the c/s/x movement. This variation creates tensions for the larger movement, and efforts to maintain a cohesive movement identity have been problematic over the long term (this will be discussed in chapter six). There are similarities as well as differences, and these are explored in the interview data.

## THE INTERVIEW DATA

In the next section of this chapter, I will present findings from my interview data, using the phases of the heroic narrative to examine the experiences of these more ordinary local activists. Pseudonyms have been assigned to protect confidentiality. In the analysis, I will introduce various forms of resistance revealed by the interview data. These forms of resistance as well as macro-level or system resistance illuminate the experience of people who are advocates working in the system, often using the services of psychiatry, yet maintaining their own resistant relations and identities as they advocate for themselves and for others.

The interview subjects in this study ranged from neophyte advocates who had "come upon" a job in the system and were initially unaware of larger movement activities, to grizzled activists with a local focus who had been involved in the national movement for up to twenty years. Most fell somewhere in between. While personal experiences may have been reframed by movement awareness, the interview narratives were deeply personal and had rarely been shared with others. In addition, they tended to be less radical and more pragmatic in their approach to psychiatry. In contrast, the public narratives and testimonies presented in conference activities and movement writings are radical stories that serve to exemplify the consumer/survivor experience and to shape a collective movement identity and purpose.

Data collected from the interviews with twelve local activists revealed numerous forms of resistance experienced by individuals who encounter the transition into psychiatric patienthood and its complex realities. Resistance can be located in terms of relative acceptance or rejection of the patient role as described by Parsons (1951); in terms of relative acceptance or rejection of the power and privilege of the physician's role (which exist in relation to the simultaneous disempowerment and discrediting of the patient role), and in terms of relative internalization or rejection of secondary deviant identity as described by Scheff (1999). In all three of these areas of analysis, individuals' experiences point to the underlying beliefs, values and goals of the movement—first at a nascent level in response to personal experience, and then with increasingly conscious, group-oriented, and activist levels of development.

At the time of the interviews, all of these individuals worked as advocates in the mental health system. As described in chapter two, they provided information, support, and intervention to help others negotiate the mental health and community systems and find ways to make choices and get their needs met. The advocates had all been diagnosed and treated for "severe and persistent mental illness." They also served on various mental health boards and committees to represent the consumer/survivor point of view, as well as on boards and committees of the Pennsylvania Mental Health Consumers' Association (PMHCA).

People who are diagnosed and treated by psychiatry ("psychiatrized") who become involved in the c/s/x movement make this choice as a consequence of their own experiences with the mental health system. (Alternatively, some people become psychiatric patients and never become involved in the movement—or, some movement leaders would say, simply don't yet recognize their own oppression.) An individual's experience of being troubled, then coming in various ways to the attention of psychiatrists who diagnosed and treated them, then moving into advocacy and into activism, were major foci of the interviews. I asked participants to describe how they had become psychiatric patients, and how they had become advocates.

As mentioned in chapter two, I was surprised to learn how many of the interviewees were currently receiving treatment from the system, even as they worked assiduously in advocacy roles to promote empowerment and self-help alternatives for their fellow mental health consumers. (The use of the terms consumer and survivor will be explored later in this chapter.)

These local advocates were not the radical anti-psychiatry activists I had been expecting. They were at once "patients," "consumers," "survivors," and "advocates." Some were medicated, some were not. Some had been hospitalized, some had not. Some had experienced forced treatment, others had not. Some had substance abuse histories, some had activist histories. Their experiences were very different, yet there were important similarities which will be described below.

## INTERVIEW VOICES AND THE SURVIVOR NARRATIVE

Analysis of the interviews reveals a correspondence of less-heroic individual experience to the phases of the survivor narrative. The individuals' experiences are more complex, more equivocal, and as could be expected, less dramatic. Their resistant practices in each of the five exemplary phases can be considered in relation to the resistance of the heroic narrative, and also to the expectations of the non-resistant, compliant patient role (as well as the doctor role) and internalization of secondary deviance. As noted above, this experience is not a step-wise process of movement or progress through phases. Instead, the phases represent different kinds of experiences that relate to aspects of involvement or identification with movement goals and activities.

### Entry into System: Trust/Distrust

First, activists commonly describe an initial acknowledgement or recognition of the need to seek help for distress or disturbance, and a willing entry into the patient role (some had been involuntarily committed, but were later convinced that their problems were caused by a psychiatric illness).

> Well, how I got in that system is I tried to commit suicide. I was going through a divorce and heavily on my addiction. Of course, I had a doctor there that did not understand about people with mental illness. Kept me there for a week or two and threw me right on the street. [Went back to the hospital], the same doctor said, we can't do anything for him except send him over to [the state hospital]. I said, well, I need help—send me there. (Jeff)

Second, they describe making an initial good-faith effort to benefit from the help given—namely, to accept a psychiatric diagnostic label, to believe the doctor's authority and expertise, and to comply with the treatment designated. These are two steps that a patient takes to move into the realm of psychiatric patienthood (psychiatrization) before the development of resistant identity—placing trust in the caregivers who define your problem, and accepting their claims to have the solution you need. Here are two examples of initial hospitalizations:

> My first hospitalization was mainly because I thought I was pregnant with God or the Devil's baby—and I couldn't decide who. So they took me to the hospital. And they put me on medicine and I was. . . I felt better . . . . So I was very lucky. And my family was very pro, Take your medication. But I still didn't believe...I didn't want to...It wasn't okay with me that I had to take this medicine forever. (Susan)

> After I had my son I was having trouble sleeping and they admitted me to the community hospital. They started me on some medication. I actually got worse instead of better. They had to admit me to a state hospital. Then I was treated as an outpatient. I had an allergic reaction to the medication, so I was admitted to the hospital and from there they took away my son and put me in my first outpatient. They diagnosed me with schizophrenia and postpartum psychosis. (Ellen)

For this patient, there is an effort to be realistic with a hint of resignation and grim humor: "And me being an in-patient and out-patient, sometimes impatient, it's like ... to do the best you can wherever you are. If you're doped up with Thorazine you do the best you can under that—and that's all you can do. And that's all you can ask of yourself, that's all anybody can ask of you, your mother, your psychiatrist, your husband, employer—anything like that." (Denise)

The advocates reveal a mixed view of the treatment system. They know that they need help, and realize that it has its less desirable aspects. They show resignation or sardonic humor. This advocate prefers to stay out of the hospital, though being there keeps her "in touch" by reminding her what it's like for those she serves in advocacy:

> And I haven't been in the hospital now for [about 10 years] and I'm thankful. But, before I was in the hospital, these last episodes, I forgot what it was like to be there and so when I had gotten in there I was like, Gee, I'm really glad I'm in here because now I'm back in touch with what it's like and now I can better hopefully serve people and stuff. But, not someplace where you want to frequent. (Denise)

One advocate, who agreed with the medical model, identified with his diagnosis ("I am bipolar") and believed his numerous hospitalizations had been "the best place for me at the time," nevertheless shows his skepticism about the psychiatrists:

> Some hospital psychiatrists are . . . short with you . . . You can't really engage them much, just out the door. And the next psychiatrist, a little bit younger, is into doing all this research on medication, you know, leading edge stuff, and willing to take the time with you and say, Hey, have you been on this, have you tried this, this, this? And it seems like, Oh my gosh, this guy sounds pretty good. He'll probably give you a placebo in the end, but, anyway . . . I'm not complaining. As far as the hospitals, I needed them. I was ill. (Joe)

These interviewees do not reject psychiatry, yet they are wary of its practices. They are ambivalent about medications, and aware of the lack of viable alternatives available within the constraints of the mental health system: "Nobody likes to be on meds. For the most part humankind does not like to take medication. I've tried to go off my meds outside of the hospital. I've tried inside of the hospital and it hasn't worked so I know that I have to take them, even though I'd rather be off of them." (Denise)

> It's like if someone has pain, we say, "Here, take an aspirin," but we don't find what the root cause of the pain is. We mask the pain, we'll diminish the pain, but we won't find out what's causing it, what's bringing it back. That's what I see the medication doing. And I take medication. There's the paradox. I take medication, because I don't have a viable alternative. (Phyllis)

When asked what the medication does for her, this advocate is realistic about why she uses it: "It keeps that intensity and that alternate consciousness at bay a bit, so that I can live my life, have relationships, work, go to the grocery store—without the inundation of symbolism and themes and intensity and the interconnections and the other-worldliness invading my everyday existence." (Phyllis)

Medication can be useful to get along in the world, for this activist, but it doesn't necessarily resolve the symptoms, which also are seen to have a certain value:

> The medications that I take, although they may be having a profound effect, I don't have a profound experience from that effect. I had a more profound experience when I didn't take them. What I take kind of takes the edge off. It doesn't resolve my depressive attitudes. It takes the edge off it though, that it's not quite so dark. I'm glad I went through some things I went through without medication because they're wonderful experiences and I cherish them, that in some circles would be called psychotic and some people would call it spiritual. To me they were just honest-to-goodness experiences that I cherish. (Henry)

The activists quoted above are describing their experience of entry into the system, and issues of trust and distrust in psychiatric treatment. These experiences correspond with the first phase of the "heroic survivor narrative." They reveal undercurrents of the themes that would be present in a more dramatic "survivor" experience, yet the activists interviewed are not emphatic about their dissatisfaction with treatment. Instead they use more indirect indicators that express a skeptical, what-can-you-do-about-it view, accepting the necessity of using a system that can help them when they choose to use it.

These individuals use subtle practices of resistance in their relationship to psychiatry, even as they are (or may be) using psychiatric care. I see these forms of resistance relating to a paradox of choice in the psychiatric system. They represent another kind of survival, of finding ways of being in the world. Often they find it necessary and desirable to use the pharmacological tools of mental health practitioners to "get along" outside (i.e., to control their symptoms adequately so they can keep a job, to avoid crises and stay out of the hospital, to act and feel as "normal" as possible). Yet, as revealed in the interviews, they continue to resist the power of the practitioners to define their "selves" and their needs. The medication is a tool to be used, it has its drawbacks, and it doesn't change their essential identity or self-determination. In fact, they emphasize their right to choose:

> If I have any problems I try to work through it prayerfully and with some close friends and family. I don't always call the doctor right away unless it would be an emergency. Because sometimes things pass. Sometimes it's a certain event that might get you flustered or . . . . Like I feel you don't call the doctor for every little thing so why should you call a psychiatrist for every little thing? (Denise)

This advocate relates an experience of early self-advocacy, of learning to make choices within the doctor-patient relationship and shape the treatment plan, deciding when to speak and still dependent on the doctor's authority:

> I wanted to get off one of my medications. So my psychiatrist, he said, 'Okay, you take it three times a day, eliminate the morning dose.' So I did and I said, it's much better, I've lost some weight, and I'm not as tired in the morning and into the afternoon, it's great. And then I noticed that I wasn't able to think as sharp or clearly and I was getting more irritable. So then, I was like, but I love these positive effects. So, I put up with that for two and a half months. Then I can't do it anymore. So then I talked to my psychiatrist and he says, 'I think you better get

back on that dose.' I says, 'Yeah, I agree.' I knew he was going to say that but I couldn't make the move without him saying it. (Denise)

When asked whether this practice of self-advocacy and speaking up in treatment assists her in advocating for others, the subject responds: "Well, that's like . . . I believe it's Pope John Paul that says, we have to evangelize ourself before we can evangelize somebody else. And also, it's been said, you can't give what you don't have. So, that's kind of like the same policy." (Denise)

Other advocates also wanted to limit their medications to function in the community: "Well, I think people knew my illness. When I got out of the hospital, I had a doctor, I was on medication. I did not want to wake up, I did not want to take a shower. But I forced myself and I went to see my doctor at the Partial Program and asked him, 'Please, because I am active across the state in advocacy, I have to keep my head cleared up.'" (Jeff)

"I have been [doing self-advocacy] all along. I have been fortunate enough to have doctors that let you tell them what you need and how much you need, and if I felt I was overmedicated, I would say so—they accepted that." (Joanne)

Thus the relationship of interviewee experiences to the first phase of the heroic survivor narrative, even in subdued form, shows evidence of a skeptical resistance to the standard "mental patient identity" or sick role, with its reliance on psychiatric expertise in defining the problem and the solution. Awareness of personal choices regarding medication adjustment, compliance, and the need to function in the community drive the negotiations of these activists with psychiatry. Neither heroic nor passive, they are active participants in the relationship. In the next section the issue of system disregard, or discrediting of personal experience, will be examined.

### System Disregard: Discrediting of Personal Realities

This activist speaks openly of her frustration about the experience of disregard, the threat of coercion, and lack of fit between her needs and their treatment:

> I was usually pretty good about taking medication that was prescribed, because I saw it as either being done voluntarily or being done forcefully, that I could go a compliant way or I could go a noncompliant way and the consequences of that, I saw, as being pretty harsh. I don't see psychiatry healing or even understanding the experiences that people go through. I think what they do is medicate it, but they don't understand it. So patienthood is very frustrating, because you're not understood. (Phyllis)

In this quote, the importance of recognizing experiential knowledge is stressed: "I guess most importantly, I try to let the people that deliver services know that they must not equate our illness with our intelligence, and that listening will be a key to their success. Because if they listen to what we have to say, then they will be able to develop the programs that will enable us to heal." (Jackie)

Talking back to psychiatry involves resistance to the psychiatric narrative. There is a dynamic of competing narratives: the narrative of the individual and the narrative of psychiatry (as represented through the individual provider or treatment team). According to the psychiatric narrative, success in treatment is often measured by "gaining insight," which involves accepting psychiatry's explanatory model of one's problem or distress; this is logically followed by "treatment compliance" which ideally leads to recovery and a resumption of as "normal" (or at least "normally deviant") a social role as possible.

Unfortunately, the psychiatric narrative also indicates that "mental illness" or "brain disease" requires life-long treatment with uncomfortable antipsychotic drugs with little chance for "recovery." This message of hopelessness and helplessness, with the promise of long-term dependency and disability implied by the labels, is internalized by some and resisted by others. This advocate describes her encounter with psychiatry's low expectations:

> They said I had schizophrenia and I would never graduate from the twelfth grade. Not only did I graduate from high school but I got my bachelors and my masters. So, it's like whenever I went back to that hospital for hospitalization there was Dr. __. And I said, "Good morning Dr. __, how are you?" I have no animosity against the guy or anything but he was wrong to judge like that. (Denise)

Then she describes her frustration with this limited view of her potential, preferring higher expectations:

> But I would tell my mom, and then we could joke about him. So, I [would like to see] providers giving consumers positions that, yeah they can do that but maybe they can do more. Because, the provider is over the consumer in such a way that sometimes they limit them unnecessarily, and the consumer will want to do more. Now granted, some consumers are happy with that and that works for them and that's good. But, like for me it wouldn't work. (Denise)

Another advocate describes how she felt when the system failed to meet her needs, but coerced her to accept their "help":

> The system was not good at that time—for me. They were not address-
> ing my problem at all. They were just telling me what they wanted me
> to do. It was not what I wanted to do at all or what I needed at all. I just
> felt coerced. I knew that I had a problem because I was aware of my
> feelings and I know what I was thinking and feeling was not right. I
> knew I needed their medication. But the rest of it I was not too fond of.
> I was hospitalized more than ten times. (Joanne)

This advocate speaks about her personal identity, her relationship with the
thoughts that make her "different" and are the basis for her psychiatric
label of "bipolar disorder":

> I know I take medicine and I have a marriage and I have a responsible
> position and I'm active in the community. But, every day my thoughts
> contain those thoughts that I had when I am labeled different. It's not
> with the intensity, it's just with subtlety. It's not pathology, but philoso-
> phy—a belief system. This is who I am. So it's like saying I'm no good.
> That's not true. Obviously not. (Phyllis)

She goes on to speak about stigma and the experience of difference: "We
honor mystics and we stigmatize crazies. And I don't know any other word
to use because that's how society looks at it—no matter how gently they try
to put it or how politically active or correct they try to put it. And I don't
feel crazy either. I feel stigmatized. I feel other-worldly. I feel that I have an
alternate consciousness." (Phyllis)

Here an activist describes her triumph, her victory of voice and self-advocacy, over a doctor who tried to keep her in the hospital against her will:

> One time [in the hospital], my time was up and my doctor was petition-
> ing for me to stay longer and I was petitioning for myself to get out so
> we went before the judge and had the hearing and stuff. And I brought
> in my shopping bag full of proof that I had collected. I explained to the
> judge, I says, "I'm on this, this is working well for me. I don't need this,
> I don't have this, I don't need this, I don't need this. And so therefore,
> I'm on the right stuff and so I should be able to go free. I'm thinking
> more clearly, I've received the help I need, blah, blah, blah, blah, blah."
> And then the doctor, he brought his case up. And then the judge, he
> agreed to let me go. And you now what, that same doctor, afterward I
> was going to get my belongings and he goes, "Looks like you won,
> [Denise]." And I says, "Looks that way." (Denise)

The third phase of the heroic narrative is especially significant. When people speak about discrediting experiences in talking about their relation to
psychiatry, there is already a resistance present in their awareness. When

psychiatric patients internalize the discrediting, there is nothing to say: they are silenced. When they talk about the discrediting, they are resisting it. For this reason, discussing the experience of discrediting and disregard already incorporates a certain amount of resistance and perhaps also action to correct the imbalance of power. In the next section, further resistance through self-advocacy, claiming the right to define one's experience, and non-compliance to treatment are explored.

### Resistant Response: Refusing Incorporation

The response to disregard and discrediting can vary in intensity. A patient might seem compliant on the surface, willing to follow the doctor's orders even if it is uncomfortable or inconvenient. Yet the reality is more complex, and the ideal of self-management comes into play. Choice and self-determination are highly valued, in contrast to the passive sick role position. This interviewee, who had spoken proudly of refusing to take medications earlier in life as a form of resistance to psychiatry, later found them useful and explained her use of medications as a personal choice: "Now, at 50-something and holding, it's a different ball game. I can say, 'Well yeah I take medicine,' but... as our body changes and as we go through the process of aging, then it's like my mind is clear because I'm taking the medication and it sort of stabilizes all my symptoms. And, it keeps me from wanting to die or to do something to myself and so it's okay." (Jackie)

The realization of active choice and self-determination marks the emergence of resistant identity within the individual-who-was-patient. This resistance occurs not just within the individual, since the patient or consumer or survivor role exists in relation to a doctor or provider. So the changes occur *in relation* to the power, authority, and expertise of psychiatry as personified within the individual's own treatment context. It can be difficult and risky to speak this resistance, to "talk back" and express a different point of view—it is often characterized by caregivers as "lack of insight" or "non-compliance," or as an actual symptom of the illness or brain disease ("aren't you grandiose").

A good patient is compliant and shows improvement by gaining insight, which means accepting the provider's view of what is wrong and what needs to be done. A bad patient who resists that view may be coercively treated or punished with restraints or seclusion "for your own good." People who feel the resistance and begin to act on it by speaking out can take different routes into the experience of "voice" in the treatment setting. Here are two different examples:

> Now the doctor that I see as an outpatient I've got to somehow con-
> vince and work with and everything to get my meds the way they should
> be. So, in the meantime I have to take it day by day and do my best each
> day even if I'm on the meds—I have to take them as prescribed even
> though I don't agree with it. Sometimes I'm an outpatient and I'll tell
> my doctor, I'll say, "I'm taking my meds as prescribed even though I
> don't always agree with it, I'm still taking these meds faithfully," and
> they're like, "Good, you do that." (Denise)

> That's when I first focused on self-help, because [some of us in the hos-
> pital] waited until everybody got to bed, at night, and then we had our
> little self-help group. That's how I really learned about self-help. And
> then this doctor found out we was doing it, he discharged two and sent
> one upstairs just to break it up, because he was scared. And that's when
> I really learned about self-help. People in the mental health profession
> was scared of it. (Henry)

One woman had held a responsible position for several years and was doing
extremely well. She came to trust her sympathetic doctor enough to reveal
some of the unusual (and personally highly-valued) beliefs she continued to
hold even while taking the medications that allowed her to keep her job and
"succeed in the world." The doctor immediately changed her diagnosis
from "bipolar disorder" (mood disorder alone) to "schizoaffective" (a combination of thought and mood disorder) since she was displaying "psychotic
thinking." She was hurt and angry about this dehumanizing experience:

> I was still the same person, everything about me was the same but I had
> told him my inner thoughts. I trusted him. I should have known better
> from past experience. So he gives me a 'worse' diagnosis. What is that
> supposed to mean? I'll tell you, they can give me any diagnosis they
> want, I'll show them I can do just fine, I can still do just as well as I am
> now. I'll show them their diagnosis doesn't mean a damn thing. (Phyllis)

It must be noted that each of the individuals interviewed had accepted the
constraints of the patient role sufficiently to succeed in a responsible social
role as an advocate in the mental health system. As mentioned, most
(though not all) were taking medication and gave credence to a certain level
of truth in their psychiatric label. Yet their interviews revealed an underlying pragmatic skepticism, indeed an active resistance to psychiatric authority that was not visible on the surface.

They described their efforts to maintain the right to define their own reality in relation to psychiatry through activities related to self-advocacy. In
addition, they worked to promote the interests of other psychiatrized persons

in relation to psychiatry, the mental health system and the community, and worked to encourage and train others to advocate for themselves. These are important aspects of the advocacy role. Helping to empower others by emphasizing self-reliance, choice and self-determination are important aspects of advocacy in mental health.

Resistance can also be enacted through what activists call "creative non-compliance." As we have seen, a person can maintain a relationship with the psychiatric system and yet maintain a separate definition of what is helpful and not helpful. At a dialogue between mental health consumer/survivors and professionals, one advocate spoke of the importance of "creative non-compliance" in finding the way to recovery. Why simply do what you are told, if the doctor does not really believe you will get better anyway?

"It is very empowering to rebel and it can be healing. Non-compliance allowed me to [recover]. If I was caught running naked through the woods, would you have paid for that "treatment"? No. Was it healing? Yes. Did I go against the rules of society? Yes." (Henry) At that same dialogue, a psychiatrist noted, "I began to understand recovery when I saw patients growing and changing even as they were still defined as ill. But I was seeing them change as individuals, as people" (Morrison 1998). This is, sadly, an important revelation, which reflects perhaps why so many patients are asking to be seen as people rather than as diagnoses.

Activists note that through creative non-compliance it is possible to test limits, take a risk, and find out what is possible. One spoke of it this way: "We have to be allowed to make our own mistakes or we will never get better. You can't protect us and help us get well." (Charles)

This activist spoke of her determination to be in control of the care she required:

> And then one time I got sick, and I had a doctor's appointment the next day. I didn't even go to the doctor's because I knew he was going to put me right in [local hospital] and that's not where I wanted to be. So I came here and I went to [another hospital] because I knew the moment he laid eyes on me that I would be in seclusion and locked up and I just didn't want it. So, I came back this way to a friendlier hospital. (Denise)

In this example, an activist made her own medication adjustment in order to be able to perform at work:

> They don't treat people with mental illness like people . . . I've had to prove myself over and over again. They had me so medicated, I was sleeping fourteen hours a day, and they were happy with that. I wanted to decrease my medication and they told me no. They told me I couldn't

do it. So I did it myself. Instead of taking three pills a day I took two. And I did it for three months and when I went back to the doctor I asked him again, "Can I decrease my medication?" (Susan)

Even with the evidence she presented (her successful self), the doctor was skeptical about the change: "I said, 'I've done it for three months and nobody has put me in jail and I sleep four hours less a day.' [He changed the prescription] but he said, if I had any symptoms break through at all, that I had to go immediately to the ER. I never had any breakthrough symptoms but I did start sleeping like ten hours a day instead of fourteen." (Susan)

In the following scenario, there are many points of contention and incredulity. The appearance of compliance is necessary to escape the spiral of authority and achieve self-determination:

> You say one thing and they may interpret it as something else, or you act one way and they might interpret something else. So you have to even know what they want you to do or say or how they want you to act so you can get out of there quicker. And then, my one doctor one time, he was increasing the dosage of my lithium so it was making my mouth dry so I was drinking a lot of water. Well, because of that [drinking a lot of water], my lithium dose was dulled down so I had to drink less water and I had to let him increase my lithium. Although I knew that wasn't a therapeutic dose, but just to get out [of the hospital]. (Denise)

She goes on to describe some of the "expert" practices that she finds impractical:

> And that's another thing. They have psychiatrists for the hospital and you get a different psychiatrist for outpatient. So, what your outpatient does the inpatient might not do. It's just kind of inconsistent. It's like, why can't your outpatient doctor come in and see you maybe or at least work [together]? They look at your records, they don't believe what you say. They look at your records from the last hospitalization, and they're not necessarily taking your word for what's going on. They'd rather believe what someone wrote about you some other time. It's a question of being taken seriously. (Denise)

This advocate has a different approach:

> Well, I didn't even negotiate. I just decided that I had to have a free mind. I just quit going and quit taking the medicine. Because, there were certain side-effects to the meds that I was taking at that time that I felt affected my thinking processes and I stayed too drowsy so I just said,

"Hey, either I'm going to fight this or I'm not." And I would not recommend to everyone to do that. And the fact was that I knew if I needed help again I could go back and get it. But, I've never really been close to any of my therapists and that, and basically I didn't trust them. And I felt that for me to do the things I needed to do, not only in the movement but for myself, my mind had to be free. (Jackie)

Another advocate described his contrasting relationship with two psychiatrists:

Well if the doctor yells at me—God bless him. Because he's apt to be reported to the right people. I had a doctor yell at me because I said I was going to sell ten thousand of those posters. Now, I didn't say I was going to sell ten thousand a day or a week . . . . So the doctor said, "You're having a delusion, you're going to sell ten thousand posters? You haven't been to college!" So I complained to the patients' rights person. (Charles)

He says later:

But see, psychiatry can change in a good way. My [other] psychiatrist, the one who helped me, he said, "I want you to be your own case manager. I want you to feel that you have as much to say, to be as knowledgeable about your own illness as some social worker, psychologist or psychiatrist." See, psychiatrists are a body of knowledge. It can be . . . domineering, taking advantage of people and enslaving people . . . and he said, "I want you to" . . . . not just, "You can." (Charles)

Activists display a range of responses to psychiatry that help them to keep one foot in the psychiatrist's office and one foot out the door. This allows for voice in the relationship, for the freedom of self-determination, and for an experience of empowerment in relation to psychiatry that is highly valued. Such relationships are made possible through challenge, negotiation or deception. All involve the use of power and choice on the part of the activist.

The power of psychiatry can be abused. Describing her experience of powerlessness during an interaction while hospitalized, this interviewee gives an eloquent and lengthy description of the loss of power that she experienced as a patient, even after years working in advocacy: "I've been an advocate for seven years. And I'm older. I know my rights, I know the commitment laws, I know a lot. And I've been with the system a long time as far as trying to make it better. And I get into a hospital a couple of years ago, and it's the hospital of my choice. . and I was agreeing to stay, I needed a time out." (Phyllis)

Even a voluntary patient, once admitted, may face a hearing in which one's right to leave the hospital must be defended against the doctor's claims that involuntary confinement is required. The "hearing officer" will ordinarily listen to the doctor's argument and the patient has the onus of proving that he or she does not need to remain hospitalized. This woman was willing to stay, but a power play was made:

> I had a young resident psychiatrist who comes in to me and says, "We're going to have a hearing for you and you can either agree to stay or I will sit in that hearing and I will not even look at you and I will talk about you like you're not even there. And I will say, this woman needs to stay here because she is a danger to herself and others." Now he says this to me when it's just the two of us, right? There's no witness to this. And I was furious. I said, "I'm agreeing to stay." And then our next confrontation I chased him down the hall calling him, "Well you little shit, you little shit!!" I was so furious that he had put me in that position of such disrespect, of such control. (Phyllis)

Reflecting on the psychiatrist's abuse of power, she states, "I would never have talked to anyone that way as a mental health advocate—and I'm on the other side. And so here I was, a mental health advocate and I was at a total loss of dignity, of control. It was such a sense of powerlessness. Because basically it would have been my word against his—and that point, who would have been believed?" (Phyllis)

She describes a moment of shared resistance and solidarity with more supportive staff:

> ". . . when one of the nurses came in, I told her what I had said and she laughed, because she knew how inappropriate he was with other people. But here he was—he was the doctor." (Phyllis)

Another encounter by this same woman reveals a similar experience of power imbalance, invasion of boundaries and disrespect: in other words, the right to define the situation. "A psychologist in the hospital, for some reason he was speaking to me in my room and it was just the two of us. And I began to feel very, very uncomfortable and did not want to answer any of his questions. I could not ask him to leave because then he'd say, 'Well, why do you want me to leave—what is your reasoning? What are you experiencing?'"(Phyllis)

A "mental patient's" actions are commonly interpreted by professionals as having significant meaning, usually pathological, not like that of a "normal" person. The power to cross boundaries, ask questions and interpret reality belongs to the staff. Freedom to control one's environment is lost in an institutional or therapeutic setting, and interactions are interpreted according to the view of the professional's own agenda. Privacy is not respected.

She goes on to describe these feelings of intrusion and exclusion:

> And at that point I couldn't talk, I couldn't tell him. I just wanted him out. And so I shut up. He was just digging, digging digging. That's not anything that was going to be healing. He needed it for his report. . . So, that's part of patienthood. That's what goes along with patienthood and the feeling of powerlessness. And you're powerless because you're not included in the process, you are swept up—you are swept up by someone's agenda and someone's process—not your own, not what's going on inside you. (Phyllis)

And, crucially, the staff controls the definition of what is required or helpful and who has the power to decide, as when hospital patients are coerced to attend group therapy: "Not what's important to you, it's whatever [they want]. Like, 'We've got to run a group, so come to this group.' That's what I mean, the groups aren't therapeutic, they're someone's idea of what's therapeutic." (Phyllis)

Another woman gave this example of unwanted programming and social control:

> There was one psychiatrist who had a daily regimen. He had each hour what you should do, get up in the morning, take a shower, eat your breakfast, go out and walk for an hour, come in and have your lunch and read something and exercise and get your housework done and exercise some more and eat your dinner and watch healthy programs and exercise some more. We called him the drill sergeant because that's the way he ran his psychiatric program. Most people, it's not what they need at all. If a person is threatening to be evicted from their house, what good is exercise going to do? And eating a healthy meal? (Joanne)

The examples cited in this section have described resistance to incorporation into the psychiatric patient identity, to the power of experts to define one's needs and experience, to a disregard of individual rights, and to the abuse of psychiatric power. In the excerpts cited, the activists have faced these challenges alone and have used creative methods of resistance to make their voices heard and create avenues for choice and empowerment. In the next section, the recognition of solidarity and shared experience will be explored.

*Solidarity: Recognizing Shared Oppression*

The fourth phase of the heroic survivor narrative involves going beyond the individual awareness of conflicting interests and the individual exercise of resistance to authority. It reveals a perception of shared awareness and development of a group consciousness—a consciousness of the value and expertise of *each other* in relation to psychiatric authority. As individuals, they had claimed the personal authority and the right to make choices in their treatment and their daily lives. Now they were finding their value to each other in providing mutual assistance and understanding of their shared realities.

This fourth phase is an awareness of peer support and self-help, a recognition of mutuality and especially valued experience, where before they had seen only the stigma of fellow mental patients whose perceptions were as discredited as their own.

The step into peer support allows for the development of group consciousness and the subsequent burgeoning of identity politics (Anspach 1979). All this is occurring in relation to the newly determined "other" of psychiatry and its practitioners, which now exist in opposition to the collective c/s/x or activated patient identity.

The woman who had described the non-therapeutic therapy groups went on to stress the value of peer interaction in the hospital setting:

> The only thing that's therapeutic in any way, shape or form is the interaction between the patients themselves. [and why do you think that is?] Because I think they're more on the same wavelength than the doctors or the support staff or the therapists, who don't have a clue. And yet, I look at people who are in the system for ten, twenty, thirty years and they are so, so, for lack of a word, so symptomatic, so unhealthy as far as . . . so psychiatrically different. And psychiatry hasn't helped a bit, not a bit. . . When people get well they get well despite psychiatry. Or they've had someone in the psychiatric process who sees them as a human being, not as an illness. And to see someone as a human being, you really have to be there . . . you really have to be there. (Phyllis)

What is helpful for people? Shared experience and recognition as a human being, reflecting the values of self-help and peer support that are basic to the movement.

The interviews revealed a resistance to psychiatry that took the form of desire for recognition and hope for change. Activists expressed an optimistic attitude and spoke of their hopes for a better system of care in the future: "The health care system for psychiatric needs has become desensitized.

They've lived in their model. Couldn't even call it a medical model anymore because it's just some kind of . . . it's a shroud. And, it's a matter of pulling them out of that shroud and see that there are some other options, some exciting things that can be done." (Joe)

While expressing their hope, the activists revealed their frustration at being treated as "less than" the so-called normal people, in spite of their expertise, their success at helping others, and their efforts at recovery:

> So why not give the consumers a shot in helping consumers? Because look at how far we've gotten with this kind of a system that we have now. Certainly, we all need to work together in various capacities, but I don't like it where it's said "Oh, a consumer can only do so much. They couldn't possibly do this, couldn't possibly do that." I've heard them talk. And, they don't really have any concept of what it's like to be inside. They think that this consumer movement with consumers running drop-in centers and stuff, consumers working, they think, "Oh, they're not going to be qualified, they're not educated enough." So, they really are against some of the consumer movement in terms of consumers being employed to help other consumers. (Denise)

Another activist describes it this way: "I guess it was the years and years of being told that I was sick because I wanted to be. Even when I almost died, they [family members] just did not support my efforts at recovery. So it was then, even before the word 'peer support' became fashionable, that I realized the strength in being with people who share common experiences." (Jackie)

The powerful effects of freedom and acceptance bring strength and motivation. Yet there is a response to a negativity that is somehow perceived as relational, a feeling of resistance to the view of some "others" who want to hold you back:

> The patients responded to [the drop-in center at the hospital] as a place to hang, a place to have coffee, a place to have cigarettes, outside the locked ward. And they felt like, yes, very comfortable there. We can move around without worrying about getting slapped in the face. And it worked out good 'til they figured out a way to get rid of me. And it's great too, the Center is still there. I did my bit. I'm in the community again and I'm better out in the community than being locked in the state hospital. (Jeff)

Acceptance and recognition of strengths are very important: "I think all of this had to do with being accepted by the people that I was working with. Also, once I realized that being sick I still hadn't lost being bright, then I felt that teacher part come out that says, Well, who better to help and to be an example for, so other people will feel a challenge that will motivate them to say, 'Well, if she can do it I can do it too.'" (Jackie)

An emphasis on recognition, on the importance of being seen and not invisible, of being valued for their abilities and successes, is a continuing theme in the interviews:

> Yes, you can plant the seed but what makes it grow? It's the people that keeps that ground moist. And I don't want them people to be forgotten about. Because, they're the ones that proves that any program would work is the consumers—they prove it works. Because they're the ones that work in it, and they're the ones that are getting, what I say, graded on it. (Jeff)

Another form of value is reflected in employment:

> The thing that makes me angry about the system right now is I see a disparity between the professionals, who get paid a lot more than the consumers and they say this out and out, but, we could hire two consumers and pay them as much as we pay one professional. I get paid less than people who really have less education than I do and don't have the years of experience that I do, in the same agency. (Ellen)

A further aspect of resistance is embodied by experiences of consciousness-raising and declaration of the value of mutual support. This process is emphasized in the heroic survivor narratives as fundamental to development and maintenance of the c/s/x movement. Much of what occurred in these advocates' lives was not directly related to the larger movement. For most of the interview participants, contact with the movement grew out of their advocacy activities, and not the other way around. In that way, we see an echo of the heroic origin stories in the interviews:

> [Interviewer: While you were engaged in these advocacy activities, did you ever feel like you were part of a larger movement?]

> I didn't know there was a national movement. I think my first exposure to national was through the National Depressive and Manic Depressive Association (NDMDA) which is medical-model based. But, that was my first exposure to people from all over the world getting together. And it's not so much what was said in the conference as what we said to each other during dinner. And that's where the feeling of a movement, or that I wasn't alone, came about. [This feeling of] connectedness, that there were people in Quebec, and there were people in Puerto Rico and in England and there were people all across the U.S. gathered

together saying the same thing over dinner. It was like, I thought I was
the only one who thought this. (Phyllis)

In attending a structured, medical-model support group, this activist
had an epiphany of connectedness and community in the unstructured, free
spaces of the gathering. [Interviewer: what kind of things were they saying
over dinner?] "We talked about our experiences and our thoughts while
people called us sick. We talked about themes of light and darkness, you
know the struggle between the forces of light and darkness. And I thought
I was the only one that was experiencing that. And all of these other people
were experiencing it also." (Phyllis)

Here the hidden transcripts (Scott 1990) of shared, taboo psychotic
thinking emerge. These experiences, which would ordinarily be seen as indicators of symptomatology and psychosis, can be safely shared and celebrated in a new supportive environment with no professionals to devalue
such thoughts by labeling them: "But nobody talks to you about that. No
psychiatrist, no therapist talks to you about that. They listen, and they say,
'Oh, that's . . .' They give it a name, delusions of grandeur, or something."
(Phyllis)

She speaks of the consciousness-raising experience of finding a shared
knowledge and world-view:

> But, they don't see the world in the same terms we were all seeing it. We
> were at a restaurant talking about different medications. We were talk-
> ing about medications and the side-effects and the funny stories about
> when we were ill, things that we would do or say. Nobody else thought
> they were funny, and, you know, people would call it manic, but . . .
> Only dressing in certain colors . . . car having a flat tire, so just walking
> away from it because it was no good any more, just giving up your car.
> And, it all made perfect sense at the time. (Phyllis)

She describes the empowerment of being together in a public place, celebrating their "craziness" without shame, and moving hidden transcripts out
into the open:

> People that were sitting around us in the restaurant, because we were
> pretty loud, were all stopping their conversations and listening to this
> incredible conversation going on. And it was like, 'Oh, we don't have
> to be ashamed of this, we don't have to be quiet. We don't have to whis-
> per it. We don't only have to say it in hospital corridors. We can say this
> in a public restaurant!' And it was very freeing and very healing. And
> from that I came away with a sense of 'I'm not alone.' (Phyllis)

About her dedication to advocacy, she explains: "Part of me wants to have fun, and part of me has a great sense of responsibility. And so part of me, even while it's a sense of responsibility, has fun with it. I go to these meetings and get into it. What would I like to do if I weren't doing this? I don't know. It's become so much a part of my life." (Phyllis)

The importance of mutuality expressed here shows similarities to the fourth phase of the heroic narrative. Even with less dramatic survival stories to share, the experience of solidarity and mutual recognition provides a powerful turning point in the development of personal and resistant identity for movement activists. In the next section, the fifth phase of politicization is explored.

### Politicization: Making Demands for System Change

In this fifth phase of the heroic survivor narrative, an individual may choose to become politically active and work for change. This politicizing awareness may develop from the sense of mutual recognition, survivor status, and collective identity. It may bring the survivor identity more strongly into the picture, with an emphasis on the experience of marginalization, disempowerment, and a negative view of abuse within the treatment system. It also may involve working toward development of alternatives and reforming the system to meet the needs of its recipients, with a more consumer-oriented focus. Yet these are not mutually exclusive identity orientations. Activists differ in their views of how to exercise power, for what reason, and with whom, when they talk about working for change.

In the following statements, issues of personal power, influence and choice are explored. This advocate is taking a strong stance in the face of actual or potential injustice and disempowerment:

> And I always go into things where, if you allow for negotiation, I'll negotiate. But I really don't know how to be intimidated. It's like no matter what your station, I'm your equal, and we may have different levels of knowledge but that doesn't make you any better or your titles or your degrees or whatever. And I always make sure that when I go I look as professional as anyone else in the field. And then I'm fortunate that I can use words well. (Jackie)

Another advocate describes an experience in which she tries to seek help in a way she feels will be more helpful than harmful. It's not easy to exercise self-determination, to direct your own treatment choices when you know what you need and others think they know better:

My reputation preceded me, of seeking after the truth and standing up for it, and standing up for others and for myself and stuff. And I know the way [local hospital] works. This one time I went to [local hospital] and I was going to go to the [receiving area of the psychiatric emergency room] and just talk to them. But they don't let you do that! The doors, there's the one door and then there's the inside doors and then you go in. Well, I'm walking inside the one door and the inside doors were locked, and so you had to ring a buzzer. . . So, this big guard was there and this other lady was there and they were about to unlock the door and I ran out the door and I ran into my car and I was like, no, no way! Because I have memories of guards dragging me and being put in seclusion for no reason at all, and just getting shot up with Haldol and given Ativan when I was told I didn't have to take it, just because I was playing my guitar. And okay, maybe it was a little loud, so close the door! No, you take an Ativan. . . So, I saw other people not being treated right, and I saw patients helping patients, and I saw myself helping patients as well as other people, and us teaming together. (Denise)

In this process of politicization, the survivor aspect may intertwine with the consumer identity, or may move beyond it. Both are activist identities and both are working for change. Also, it is crucial to recognize that people move and shift along this consumer/survivor continuum over time in both directions, as illustrated by the interviewees and in the larger movement community. It is not a step-wise process of unidirectional change.

## TERMINOLOGY AND LABELS

As discussed in chapter three, a simplistic dichotomized analysis of anti-psychiatry survivors and co-opted drug-popping consumers is inadequate to convey the complex political and personal realities of these activists and their movement. The survivor and consumer identities are not separate entities; they can occur simultaneously or serially in the same person. However, this topic is often a matter of debate: what do members call themselves, and does it matter?

I asked about these terms in the interviews and received some interesting responses about the terminology of consumer/survivor/ex-patient, and the right to self-definition:

I don't even think it's ever been properly defined. As far as a label, I don't think we have a label for it. I think we keep defining it in terms of the medical model. Mental health consumers, psychiatric survivors, ex-patients, it's not in terms of my experience. And if we all reframed the experience, we may find other words. Teacher, mentor, maybe

there's something to be offered there that we haven't even begun to explore. (Phyllis)

Another advocate prefers the term consumer to describe her experience:

> Survivor to me sounds like you've been in a concentration camp. Can't
> stand that. Ex-patient, I don't like patient. I do not like patient. And ex-
> patient to me sounds like, well, you're too optimistic that you're never
> going to go back in. And, consumer, the first time I heard consumer I
> said, "What in the hell's that?" But, I like that and I like it more and
> more. You are a consumer of services. You can get up and you can go
> and you can get treatment wherever. I don't feel like I should be
> ashamed that I'm a mental health consumer. (Ellen)

This long-term advocate considers the instrumental meaning of the changing labels:

> Well, consumer, a bunch of us developed [that label] to get rid of the
> stigma of patient, ex-patient, client, okay. Now, after the consumer has
> been in existence now maybe for fifteen, twenty years, now they're
> upset with that. What do you want to be called? Now at this time,
> 2000, the younger group should come up with another thing and put it
> through the system. Us old timers were glad consumers was developed
> to get away from ex-patient or client. (Jeff)

This respondent reveals his insight into the complexity of the term consumer and the underlying disempowerment of its current use for "recipients
of mental health services":

> I know people that by definition are consumers, but they're not on med-
> ical assistance so they don't consider themselves consumers. Consumers
> is . . . To me, that definition has become to mean the helpless, the peo-
> ple that are on disability, on SSI [Supplemental Security Income] in par-
> ticular. And I've talked to people that take medications but they're not
> consumers. They go to therapy but they're not consumers. They see psy-
> chiatrists personally but they're not . . . It's replaced welfare. I think
> that's its designation. (Henry)

And this response reflects a more philosophical view about labels:

> Well, having been so used to wearing so many labels, it really doesn't
> make me any difference. However, when I present [at conferences]
> where I'm talking about myself, my choice of word is survivor. When
> you allow yourself to get uptight about the labels, then you get locked

into where you can't go forward. So you know, I don't have to own the
labels just because someone gives them to me. (Jackie)

These two activists have different views but both see the power of labels to
define reality, and place an emphasis on the need to change the perception
of "mental illness" and treatment, and to define it on their own terms: "I
would like to see us drop the whole medical thing and see where we can go
with the other, with the philosophical, the metaphysical, with the psychological. We have this political animal called the DSM-IV [Diagnostic and
Statistical Manual]. And that's political. And that's how everyone is gauged.
But that's not by us, that's by psychiatrists. It needs to be by us." (Phyllis)

> I think the problem is, in the public's mind, not enough is done to erase
> the stigma. I think that too many articles are written about killers and
> too much public knowledge when people commit crimes, their mental
> health history is revealed. I just saw the movie, *Girl Interrupted*. And I
> thought, now that didn't happen to me when I was in a state hospital.
> In fact, I got slapped, and held down, and needles were shot in my arms,
> and I was tied to a bed! I think those are dramatic things, but, it also
> shows what's reality. (Ellen)

The process of politicization ranges from seeing the issues in terms of power
and definition, to taking action and working to create change through various means. There were varied responses in the interviews related to personal involvement in the movement and making change in that way. Not
everyone involved in advocacy at the personal, local or regional levels is also
participating in national movement activities:

> I've been real hesitant to go on a national campaign, or even network-
> ing on a national level. I don't know why. I don't want to say it's futile,
> but I guess I don't have a lot of expectations or hope for it. I don't think
> there's a lot of understanding for what I'm saying. I honor those that are
> able to make inroads and changes through the political process or the
> activist process, but it doesn't pull my heart. Getting a voice, and get-
> ting a voice for my experience, that is what pulls my heart. (Phyllis)

Yet other advocates found their strength through participation at the larger
levels:

"I tell you when I went to the first national conference that's where I
met all my contacts. Didn't know anybody. I got off that bus, met _____, I
met them all there. And I just shook hands, I was very outspoken to get to
know people in the movement. That's where I'm at." (Jeff)

"[I was] drawn into it, asked to participate. Went to my first consumer conference, and that was quite an experience. It was an opportunity for me to feel included, if you will, in the bigger picture. And that's when I met ___ and she became my mentor from that point on. And I guess my need was to become like her." (Jackie)

A sense of creating change, though very slowly over time, is eloquently expressed by this advocate, who is able to see that he has made a difference through working with the c/s/x movement:

> I was part of the voice changing the system. It was hard work. When you seen a little bit, like a little dust particle of change of the movement, well, we are making some progress. If I could see just a dust of progress, that means it's working. Cause you're not going to get a big chunk. You have to nibble at it. In the years that you nibble at it, then you get big chunks. But it took us, where the movement is today, it took us a good twenty years to get where we're at today. (Jeff)

## REVISITING THE HEROIC SURVIVOR NARRATIVE

The five-phase framework of the heroic survivor narrative corresponds with the experience of ordinary activists. Each of these phases represents opportunities for resistance, and individuals will make their own choices about how to enact these moments in their personal lives. A recognition of the underlying connections between the survivor narrative and everyday psychiatric c/s/x experience allows further understanding of the importance of this narrative to the movement at large.

The survivor experiences exist in a range of intensity, from high drama to muted skeptical observations. Yet even muted, their presence in various forms is evident as a force, and as a vehicle, for developing resistant behaviors and identities at various points in the survivor narrative. Betrayal of hope and trust, the experience of disregard and discrediting, refusal to incorporate psychiatric labels and expectations, all these experiences were described and resisted by the activists interviewed. Their further experiences of solidarity and mutual support, their varying degrees of politicization and choices of fields for action, demonstrate the commonality of experience among people who have been psychiatrized and choose to resist the power and authority of psychiatry and advocate for others.

In the larger movement, these themes of resistance are re-enacted and emphasized in group settings that build collective identity and shared experience. Compelling personal stories are told regularly at conferences and support group meetings. Witnessing and testimonies are published in books, magazines and on the web. They reveal the same framework. Based on the interview analysis and comparison with more dramatic (and sometimes legendary) public stories of survival, it becomes clear that the mechanisms and messages are similar in the development of resistant identities along the various individual paths to activism and advocacy.

The themes that emerge from the interview data both illuminate and challenge the "accepted" (yet still energetically contested) currently-used categories of experience such as consumer, survivor, ex-patient, and person-in-recovery that have led to controversies and splits in the movement as well as attacks by outsiders. At the same time, when examined in relation to the stories told by the long-term movement activists and leaders, and to the established collective identities of the movement, these themes reveal important underlying continuities that have enabled the movement itself to survive—as its members find a fundamentally shared experience (disregard, damage, oppression) that goes beyond the differences to make possible a shared identity with common goals and purposes.

The survivor narrative which follows the form outlined above is a vital part of the movement identity. These narratives are re-enacted at public conference events each year. Telling these stories creates solidarity and helps to form collective identity, as members reframe their own experiences in this narrative form and celebrate their own survival along with their peers.

# Chapter Five

# Talking Back through the Larger Movement: Campaigns and Initiatives

> The only purpose for which power can be rightfully exercised over any member of a civilized community, against his will, is to prevent harm to others. His own good, either physical or moral, is not a sufficient warrant.
> —John Stewart Mill, 1859 (quoted in *The Rights Tenet,* Spring 2001:22)

## INTRODUCTION

The movement goals of Breaking the Silence and Ending Psychiatric Oppression have been explored historically in chapter three; their development through expressions of individual resistance were described in chapter four. The purpose of this chapter is to illustrate the expression of movement goals in the campaigns and initiatives that are part of the everyday life and the special events of the movement. A sampling of movement activities reveals a variety of efforts and strategic choices that work toward the same goals and express the same themes, related to coming to voice and talking back to psychiatry within the solidarity of the larger movement.

## MOVEMENT LEADERSHIP

By observing movement activities and interactions, I soon found that there is no national structure with centralized leadership. The leaders are the people who are most visible in the movement, who dedicate themselves to setting the agendas and promoting action among the members. They are important as organizers, catalysts and role models for other members, both long-term and newly identifying with the movement. The major leaders of today have been active in the movement for up to 30 years, including Ted Chabasinski, Judi Chamberlin, Pat Deegan, George Ebert, Janet Foner, Leonard Roy Frank, Jay Mahler, David Oaks, Joseph Rogers, Don Weitz, Sally Zinman, and others. These individuals embody and personify the origins, the splits, the continuity, the energy, the dedications, the strengths and the weaknesses of the movement.

Their stories are legendary (their personal survival stories, their interactions with each other over the years, even their deaths) and create the mythology of the movement: its past as well as its present. These stories have been published in various forms, enough to be considered public knowledge, though they are public knowledge only within the circles of the movement and to a few researchers.

The leaders of the most visible organizations are among the nationally recognized leaders as well. The National Empowerment Center in Lawrence, Massachusetts (www.power2u.org), is led by Dan Fisher, M.D. and Laurie Ahern. The National Mental Health Consumers' Self-Help Clearinghouse in Philadelphia (www.mhselfhelp.org) was started by Joseph Rogers. Support Coalition International (SCI) (www.mindfreedom.org) in Eugene, Oregon, led by David Oaks (and formerly Janet Foner), is the group that started publishing the *Dendron News* (now known as *MindFreedom Journal*) in 1988 after the demise of the *Madness Network News*. SCI is a loosely organized coalition of about one hundred groups in the U.S. and around the world who communicate through the Internet, phone and written communication to organize activities and support each other in their efforts to protect rights and resist forced treatment by psychiatry.

All of these groups, and many others, use their influence and visibility to develop ideas and information, and to focus on local issues and services. Some of the most dynamic leadership, veteran and emerging, also resides in important local organizations such as The Alliance in upstate New York, the California Network of Mental Health Clients, and the West Virginia Mental Health Consumers' Association, to mention only a few. Leaders in these groups use their considerable energy on local issues, and also have an impact on the larger level at annual conferences and demonstrations, joining others by working behind the scenes on focused campaigns and strategy development. Leadership in this movement evolves from action and inspiration, not form or rank. C/s/x leaders are working from the power of their resistance and their goals for change, as well as their personal energy and ability to energize others.

Movement leaders who work in the professional fields of law, psychiatry and psychology are also an important part of the movement. They are active in some of the groups mentioned above. They also take leadership roles through their work with dissident professional groups that cross the boundaries between professional providers and consumer/survivors such as the National Association for Rights Protection and Advocacy (NARPA) (www.narpa.org), the International Center for the Study of Psychiatry and Psychology (ICSPP) (www.icspp.org), and the Bazelon Center for Mental Health Law (www.bazelon.org) Some of these individuals, such as Tom Behrendt, Ron Bassman (2001), Peter Breggin (1991, 1997, 1999), David Cohen (Cohen & Breggin 1999), Loren Mosher (1996, 1999, 2002) and Susan Stefan (2000), have devoted their professional lives to the movement. They face the risks of stigma and discrediting in their professional lives, due in some cases to personal experiences of psychiatrization, as well as their deep and lasting personal connection to movement issues and concerns. Other joint efforts include cross-disability alliances with disability rights activists such as the American Association of People with Disabilities (AAPD) (www.aapd.dc.org) and *Mouth* (www.mouthmag.com).

With the leadership that I have described, as well as local leadership throughout the U.S. and around the world, the ongoing campaigns of the movement have been negotiated, set, and put into action. The campaigns are long-term and open-ended, since the goals of increasing voice, choice, reducing harm, and increasing alternatives for people in the psychiatric system are not goals that are easily met or reach an endpoint. In the next section, I will describe some of the campaigns that I have witnessed in action during my participation in the movement.

## LARGER MOVEMENT GOALS

Movement activists all over the United States (and other parts of the world including Australia, Brazil, Canada, Columbia, Denmark, France, Germany, India, Israel, Netherlands, New Zealand, Norway, Pakistan, Palestine, and the United Kingdom) are engaged in an ongoing campaigns related to instances of psychiatric abuse, proposed changes in commitment laws and public policy, new developments in pharmaceutical research and in psychiatric treatment. Activists are watching for opportunities for representation like President Bush's New Freedom Commission, the White House Conference on Mental Health, and the *Surgeon General's Report on Mental Health*. They also monitor and respond to negative propaganda about people labeled with psychiatric diagnoses. (Such messages are often used by enemies of the movement to magnify fear and public concern that can be leveraged into more support for actions to restrict the rights of psychiatrized persons in the community.)

Consumer/survivor/ex-patient activists amplify the personal aspects of resistant identity and talking back by taking their claims and grievances into the larger public arena. The campaigns and ongoing strategies focus on central movement issues of voice and representation, exposing and challenging expert psychiatric knowledge and practice, promoting and developing alternatives to traditional treatment, and prevention of human rights abuses such as forced treatment.

Keeping abreast of these issues requires constant vigilance and monitoring of information sources. This activity is greatly enhanced by the use of the Internet. Newspapers, medical journals, websites, etc. are monitored every day. Many people are involved in these activities with a few central nodes of information flow, supported by dozens of group and individual websites (a sample is available in Appendix B). There is also active participation in topical listservs, members of which can be galvanized into action when needed.

Little of this activity is seen by members of the public or mentioned in the media. Yet the activities are effective and consequential. Some of the best recent evidence for the movement's effective influence can be seen in the increasingly virulent attacks on the movement by two of its most public opponents, labeled "extremist psychiatrists" by David Oaks: Doctors E. Fuller Torrey and Sally Satel, described later in this chapter.

Many of the movement's activities are responses to actions performed by others, mobilizing activity to speak out for individual rights and assure the presence of the voices of people who have been psychiatrized. "Nothing about us without us" is an important slogan of the movement and is a sort of backdrop to all its activities. The struggle for voice and representation, fighting for attention in the face of discrediting polemics and disregard, and discovering creative new areas for action are all important to the movement.

## A DIVERSIFIED FRAMEWORK

When sampling the strategies, tactics, and campaigns of the c/s/x movement—the "public" aspects of talking back—it is important to note that the movement is not centralized or organized in a top-down fashion, and there is no national organization. Instead, the major leadership groups I have mentioned provide a core for the diverse coalition that brings focus and energy for collective action. Movement activities are diverse and include hundreds of local and regional groups and individuals who consider themselves activists and who relate to a collective identity of "the c/s/x movement."

The movement's existence and growth are maintained by this valued relationship, with accommodation for differences as well as shared beliefs.

Recognizing and nurturing a diverse constituency is a challenging way to manage a movement. Differences and schisms have historically caused great turmoil, feuds and personal suffering. Leaders have had longstanding disagreements about whether to pursue or accept funding from the federal government, state and local governments, even pharmaceutical companies. Recent efforts to overcome such differences and become more inclusive while maintaining core values have allowed the movement to respond with more unity, flexibility and strength to threats from the outside, including forced treatment programs, funding cuts and challenges to rights protection. In the face of these challenges, leaders and members are learning to overcome their historical differences and rediscover common themes that underlie the movement's existence and long-term continuities. Over the long term and into the present, the primary goals of the movement (and some representative campaigns) can be characterized as follows:

## GOAL 1. SPEAKING OUT TO BREAK THE SILENCE ABOUT PSYCHIATRIC OPPRESSION AND ABUSE: "THERE ARE MORE OF US THAN YOU THINK."

### Voice and Empowerment

Movement activists place great emphasis on encouraging people who have been psychiatrized to find their voices, to speak up about their experiences in the mental health system. Not only does this empower individuals, it empowers the movement as well. Since the earliest days, the c/s/x movement has worked to provide spaces for open conversation and mutual support, emphasizing that the voices of the psychiatrized must be heard to expose the truth about abuse and suffering in the mental health system.

Breaking the silence includes people telling their stories, in the same sense as the witnessing and testimony of those who have been silenced by political regimes or religious persecution. When these stories are shared by those with similar experience, or heard by those who have been unaware, another truth ("our truth") is exposed. There are many means for fulfilling this goal by spreading the word; only a few will be presented here.

As described in chapter three, the *Madness Network News (MNN)* was the major instrument for developing individual awareness and community action in the early days of the movement. *MNN* invited people to speak out, and also exposed formerly-hidden psychiatric knowledge about diagnosis and treatments. Other publications, most notably *Dendron* and *MindFreedom Journal,* have continued these initiatives. Raising voices and demystification were important goals for the early movement and their importance continues today.

## Using New Technologies

Recently, the Internet provides a new kind of madness network (see Appendix B). Internet sites play a major role in building, maintaining, and motivating movement identity and action. Websites and listservs that provide a means for telling personal stories and debating the pros and cons of psychiatric treatment have proliferated in the last several years. These sites allow people to reveal their histories with psychiatry, post them on the web, and respond to each others' stories. They post a variety of dissenting views and links to information from many sources that may be useful to movement members. Education and self-expression, along with peer support, are important components of advocacy.

Because sites are open, they also invite debate; people who feel they have benefited from psychiatry can disagree with the positions taken by the more radical participants. Professionals also participate; some assert their authority and superior wisdom, others take a more radical view. In this process, a conversation is possible that was not occurring before. A free space (Groch, 2001) is provided for dissenting voices to create oppositional consciousness, and the word can spread widely in the free access provided by these sites. People develop their stories and their movement identities in relation to each other on the Internet and in their local communities as they locate each other and work to create change in their communities and the mental health industry.

"Peoplewho.org" is a website that was started by Sylvia Caras as an early listserv for "people who." The words in the site name show the emphasis on "people first" language. This usage emphasized being seen as a person, not as a diagnosis. The "peoplewho" site was created for people who heard voices, saw visions, and in other ways were different enough to have come to the attention of psychiatry. This successful site has expanded greatly over the years. It now has branches for specialty concerns, including social responsibility, actmad, social accountability, MadGrrls, grassroots, TwoHats (for "people who" who also work in the mental health field) voice-hearers, and many others. It also includes geographically focused topic areas for discussion and support organized by state or region, and has introduced a Spanish language list ("De-Locos") among many others lists, both public and private. This listserv is a valuable resource for connection with other "people who" have had similar experiences of difference of various kinds.

The website for Support Coalition International (mindfreedom.org) also provides multiple forums for discussion, including "noforce" for discussions and development of campaigns against forced treatment, and "healnorm," a wide-ranging discussion group based on an earlier campaign to "heal normality naturally" which challenged assumptions about "normality" by labeling aspects of normal behavior as strange and undesirable. The "Ten Warning Signs of Normality" free self-test, for instance, includes:

> Warning sign #5, "Boring: Your conversations, life and living space are dull and boring, and your lawn is always manicured no matter what. In the more advanced stages you have much inner 'lifelessness' and 'flat affect'—in other words, you are one of the 'walking dead.' Your psychiatric label is "hyper-inactivity."

> Warning sign #7, "Gullible: You believe that the doctor always knows best, that the media is telling the truth (major newspapers always print the facts, right?) and that the medical model of 'mental illness' has been proven scientifically. Your diagnosis is "normal naiveté disorder" (Foner n.d., SCI).

This "public service announcement" has been widely distributed as a poster, to be snowballed with permission. Regularly on sale at regional and national conferences, it provides an example of the wry humor in combination with a call to action, often used by the movement to make its point about taking voice and seeing psychiatric wisdom in new ways. The poster concludes with an invitation:

> Don't Panic: If you have two or more of these signs within any lunar cycle, it is not too late. Join SCI, read *Dendron News,* support one another, get out into nature, and especially take action to stop psychiatric oppression before serious persistent "normality" sets in. For more information, write [space for contact information] (Foner n.d., SCI.).

Newer versions of this poster contain the SCI website address (www.mindfreedom.org) which stimulates significantly more response and information flow for SCI than the "snail mail" contact address of the past.

More organized methods for collecting and telling personal stories are in process in various parts of the country. For example, Pennsylvania Mental Health Consumers Association (www.PMHCA.org) has been collecting stories on videotape at its annual conferences. Mindfreedom.org recently introduced a specific oral history site for "telling our stories" as a political act, with narratives that reveal personal truths and promote the goals of the movement:

> The Support Coalition International (SCI) Oral History Project involves collecting stories from psychiatric survivors, consumers, and ex-patients about their experiences in the mental health system: powerful stories of recovery, survival, resistance, and self-determination. There are plenty of stories circulating about people labeled with psychiatric disabilities who have "improved" or even "recovered," as a result of a strict diet of medication and perhaps a little therapy. Less is heard about people who either did not use mental health services or who now reject that system, and who have fought through tough times, survived and are now functioning well, possibly even better than ever. Much can be learned from these people about the nature of survival, recovery, and well-being (http://www.mindfreedom.org/histories.shtml).

The website at www.Mindfreedom.org is a centrally important site for organizing, political action and awareness. It provides information about the movement and exposes abuses in the psychiatric and pharmacological industries. This site has links for Urgent Action, Current Campaigns, a Mad Market for books and videos, and a sign-up for email alerts with an archive of earlier alerts and press releases. To quote its mission statement, "Support Coalition International will take leadership in vitalizing the mind freedom movement by uniting groups in a cooperative spirit, celebrating empowering emotional support, and launching human rights campaigns that activate a wide diversity of the public. Our mutual support gives us the power to speak the truth!" (http://www.mindfreedom.org/about.shtml)

Support Coalition International also publishes a print journal, *Mind Freedom*. The journal is considered to be the descendant of *Madness Network News* though it has evolved into a magazine format that has recently been published about once a year, illustrating the new reliance on electronic media in the movement. However, SCI also emphasizes its historical origins:

> The roots of Support Coalition International go deeply into the psychiatric survivors' liberation movement itself, which came directly out of civil rights ferment of the late 1960s and early 1970s. The description "psychiatric survivors" is used by individuals who identify themselves as having experienced human rights violations in the mental health system. In the past thirty years, many grassroots groups working for those labeled with mental disabilities sprang up nationally and internationally.

They also make clear their more radical positioning on the activist continuum, and emphasize their growth through the 1990s:

> However, since the mid-1980s many of these groups became primarily federal or state funded, and therefore their independent human rights political activity is limited. In late 1988, leaders from several of the main national and grassroots psychiatric survivor groups decided an independent coalition was needed, and Support Coalition International was formed. The first action of SCI was a counter-conference and protest in New York City in May 1990, at the same time as the American Psychiatric Association huge annual meeting. The initial coalition had thirteen organizations. Today, Support Coalition International unites more than one hundred grassroots sponsoring organizations in fourteen nations (http://www.mindfreedom.org/about.shtml).

The site "antipsychiatry.org" serves as another excellent example. This is a personal site, created by Douglas Smith of Topeka, Kansas, who was diagnosed with schizophrenia and started the site to tell his own story and to voice his objections to psychiatric treatment, while inviting others into the conversation. This site includes lengthy debates between the webmaster (Smith) and psychiatrists who are trying to debunk his position, with supportive comments interspersed by other visitors to the site who express their various views. It also features extensive writings by various authors and experts who are challenging the authority and practices of psychiatry:

> The Antipsychiatry Coalition is a nonprofit volunteer group consisting of people who feel we have been harmed by psychiatry—and of our supporters. We created this website to warn you of the harm routinely inflicted on those who receive psychiatric treatment and to promote the democratic ideal of liberty for all law-abiding people that has been abandoned in the U.S.A., Canada, and other supposedly democratic nations (http://www.antipsychiatry.org/).

Other examples of individual sites include the Lunatics Liberation Front (LLF) in Canada (http://www.walnet.org/llf/) and http://psychiatrized.org in Alaska. LLF is a wonderfully imaginative site by Irit Shimrat, author of *Call Me Crazy: Stories from the Mad Movement* (1997). The opening page of this site is provocative and gives great insight into the movement, which really must be experienced to be understood:

> LLF is an information network whose main subject is alternatives to psychiatry. Its aim is to promote the liberation of people who have been

or are in danger of being labelled mentally ill—those who go nuts or get too angry, too "high" or too miserable for their own and/or other people's comfort—from:

- the belief that we have incurable diseases and are not responsible for our own behaviour;
- the expectation that we cannot hope to control our own lives;
- people's expectations that we will behave badly;
- psychiatric hospitals and wards where we learn to hate and doubt ourselves;
- treatments that damage our bodies, brains and minds....

I believe crazies need to be in touch with each other and with sympathetic people who haven't been caught yet. Internationally, mad people are organizing and spreading the word about alternatives to medical treatment for emotional problems (http://www.walnet.org/llf/).

Irit's site expresses the essence of oppositional consciousness, using a combination of humor and outrage at the contradictory assumptions and practices of psychiatry. She includes the messages of voice, alternatives, rights protection, abuse, and peer support in her internet message of solidarity and freedom.

Most of these sites include multiple links to each other and to other sites (including more conventional mental health sites, government sites, sites about legal rights, about conferences, etc.). In this way they provide a natural network that can be accessed by anyone from a personal computer or in the public library. Once someone has referenced this network, the possibilities for connection and information are open-ended. This informal, voluntary information outreach campaign is very effective for the movement. It provides a forum for expression of grievances, witnessing, debate, consciousness-raising, and constructive change.

## GOAL 2. SPEAKING OUT TO CHALLENGE THE AUTHORITY OF PSYCHIATRY AND ITS ABUSE OF POWER: "SILENCE IS COMPLICITY"

Grievances about unjust treatment, coercion, and abuse have been framed in various ways. A human rights frame was dominant in the early years of the movement. Later, more specific efforts to protect mental patients' rights were emphasized. More recently, a return to the human rights frame has accompanied an effort to cross boundaries with other rights groups, particularly disability rights, and crossing international boundaries. The Internet, which seems a very private site of contention even as it is shared by many individuals, also serves as a vehicle for mobilization of campaigns in both the private and public arenas.

### Human Rights Alerts

The existing network described above serves as a vast source of public pressure when a human rights campaign alert appears. In one example, a woman was the object of coercive treatment with psychotropic drugs, even against her family's objections. A family member contacted David Oaks at SCI, who sent out an alert bulletin with detailed information on the situation, including email and telephone contacts for the director of the agency ordering the treatment. Within a short time, the agency was deluged with hundreds of calls and emails protesting her situation. As a result of this intervention, the treatment was discontinued and the woman returned home.

This sort of unexpected intervention is very powerful, as it effectively exposes hidden practices to public view. The woman in question was so grateful for the enthusiastic response to her plight, she became an activist in a movement she had never heard of, and her victory story was featured in the newsletter. These triumphant victory stories are an effective part of the movement, as they convey the success that can be achieved when large numbers of people are moved to speak out for others, challenging the authority of the mental health system to overrule the rights of individuals in the name of unwanted "treatment." These stories are rarely heard outside of movement circles.

### Rescue and Safety

Another rescue aspect of the movement must remain hidden, as it involves risky illegal activity for protection of rights. As involuntary outpatient treatment in the community becomes more prevalent in many states, the development of an "underground railroad" has been suggested to help people leave the state where their rights have been violated by a court order to forced outpatient drugging. A network of safe houses and transportation assistance was developed and may now be in operation, but I have not followed up on this effort at rights protection, so as not to place it at risk. I mention it because it alerts us to the importance of human rights issues in the movement, and the very real fact that life and death situations are faced by people in the psychiatric system. These folks are not just playing around. The knowledge that a person is not alone, but has a network of allies who will be available in case of hospitalization or coerced treatment, is central to the movement. The early days of abandonment behind locked doors are being emphatically reversed.

It is not easy to convey the depth of commitment and the seriousness of the movement in and for people's lives. Early in my research, I was traveling to a national alternatives conference and sat next to a woman of apparent means. When she asked about my destination, I explained briefly about the movement of mental health consumer/survivors. She responded, "Well, can't they just change analysts?" When I explained further, she remarked, "If this kind of problem exists, it should be exposed, like on Oprah." Public awareness is so limited, and so framed by the psychiatric and demonized-madperson narratives, it is a real challenge for the movement to be taken seriously except by people who are already aware of the issues and choose to adjust their interpretation into the movement injustice frame.

### Public Campaigns and Demonstrations

A recent high-profile campaign involved two men at New York's Pilgrim State Psychiatric Center who were subjected to involuntary electroshock treatments. Their court hearings were publicized by movement activists, through Support Coalition news briefs and New York activist networks. The press was contacted by the movement and became interested, particularly the *New York Post,* which closely followed the story. Protests were held to draw attention to the situation and make it clear to the authorities that these treatment decisions were under public scrutiny.

The eventual outcome was discontinuation of forced shock, and also the resignation of one New York State mental health advocate who was forbidden to become involved in the protest, so quit her job in the face of such an extreme conflict of interest. In addition, the furor attracted the attention of a New York State legislator who initiated an investigation of the use of shock in New York State hospitals. This was a nearly ideal case in which talking back worked: intervention was successful, media attention was drawn to movement issues and abusive treatment, and policy changes became a possibility. It was not completely ideal because during the process, one of the men received more forced shock when the restraining order was overturned by a judge during the proceedings (he had already been subjected to a series of forty involuntary electroshocks against his expressed wishes).

Electroshock is one of the ongoing issues for the movement. Efforts to ban ECT entirely have been a source of internal strife; the less radical position of objecting only to *forced* shock is seen a sort of compromise position. Nevertheless, the damaging effects of electroshock, especially memory loss, and the lack of truly informed consent are the subject of a continuing campaign ("The Right to Remember") and the subject of another important movement website, www.ect.org. Recently there has been interest in renewing the "Shock Doctor Roster" (a list of doctors who administer ECT, which had its origins in the *Madness Network News*), to raise public awareness of these issues.

Recurrent sites of public demonstration for the movement are the annual conventions of the American Psychiatric Association and the annual Mad Pride festivities occurring every summer on Bastille Day (July 14th). Other demonstrations are aimed at particular sites. In 1998 I participated in a protest with more than 150 others at Metropolitan State Hospital outside of Los Angeles. The march had been scheduled to coincide with the "Alternatives '98" conference in nearby Long Beach, to protest the abuse of children at the hospital. According to Ted Chabasinski's article in the *Dendron News*:

> Children at Metro are frequently put into five-point restraints (tied to a bed with leather straps at their wrists, ankles, and waist) for the slightest infraction. The hospital's own statistics…showed that restraints are used hundreds of times a month. The kids are heavily drugged and almost never get to go outside their locked wards. Most belong to ethnic minorities, and some are as young as nine years old (Winter 98/99:18).

Ted Chabasinski has a special interest in children's rights and psychiatry. He spent his youth in a state institution, and is a survivor of forced electroshock he received as an experimental subject at six years of age. He was one of the early movement organizers in California and is now an attorney in Berkeley, working to protect the rights of the psychiatrized. Marching with Ted and the others at Metro State was a powerful experience of unity and purpose. It rained all afternoon, but the marchers stayed in front of the hospital gates with soggy picket signs and called out to cars passing by, marching to call attention to the abuse of children inside the gates. We traveled together in two buses with our signs and ponchos and that was a day of solidarity I will not forget.

Participating in demonstrations brings members of the movement together, and creates the solidarity and sense of purpose that motivates people to continue their identification with the movement, as well as express their grievances. Typical protest signs include Psychiatry Kills, No Forced Treatment, Silence = Complicity, Ban ECT, You Bet Your Ass We're Paranoid, Stop Forced Drugging, Mad Pride, and Forced Psychiatric Drugging Is Tyranny. Here is the description of a counterprotest to "break the silence about forced psychiatry" at a federally-sponsored "Walk the Walk" march in Washington on May 2, 1998.

David Oaks wrote this report of the event:

> The Clinton Administration expected their $200,000 public relations
> event . . . would present a nice united front to promote the mental
> health system. They hoped that thousands of people would gather in
> Freedom Plaza a few blocks from the White House, and cheer on the
> psychiatric establishment. . . One Counterprotest, sponsored by
> Support Coalition, was led by survivors of human rights violations in
> psychiatry [who] used guerrilla theater to make our 'point.' We hoisted
> lots of big fake hypodermic needles onto tall wooden poles to protest
> force drugging. We had ten hypos that were five feet long, and one huge
> ten-foot prop hypo dubbed 'Big Bertha'. . . We especially targeted the
> increased use of forced outpatient psychiatric drugging (*Dendron
> News,* Winter 98/99,10).

Another participant described the scene: "Most of us held home-made signs
that reflected our individual feelings about psychiatry: 'Psychiatry is not
health care,' 'Stop forced psychiatric drugging,' 'Bet your ass we're paranoid,' 'Walk the walk for lives ruined by psychiatry,' 'NAMI & NIMH promote psychiatric assault,' 'Keep your laws off my body and mind,' and
others" (*Dendron News,* Winter 98/99, 11).

At the same event, Justin Dart, a leader of disability rights activism,
gave a speech in support of the counterprotest. His remarks illustrate the
growing effort to unite the two movements "across disabilities":

> People with psychiatric disabilities are still among the most oppressed
> people in the world. Millions are denied employment, health care, hous-
> ing . . . forced to take drugs and other treatments in violation of their
> most fundamental constitutional rights. . . I propose that we of the dis-
> ability communities unite with all who love justice to lead a revolution
> of empowerment. We have unique knowledge, unique experience, and
> therefore unique responsibility to lead a revolution, to create a culture
> that will empower every single individual including all people with psy-
> chiatric disabilities, to live his or her god given potential for self-deter-
> mination, productivity and quality of life (*Dendron News,* Winter
> 98/99,13).

In the *Dendron News* and other movement publications, the reader is bom-
barded with news of activism and organizing activities in the U.S. and
around the world. However, these activities are rarely featured in the mainstream press so the public is not informed about the issues, or about the
c/s/x movement. Thus the movement experiences simultaneous visibility
and invisibility: visibility and effectiveness at the policy level, promoting
self-help and consumer-run programs around the nation; invisibility at the

public level except for people who are already "insiders" to movement activities or are acting to counter its influence.

## GOAL 3. SPEAKING OUT TO INFLUENCE PUBLIC MENTAL HEALTH POLICY: "NOTHING ABOUT US WITHOUT US"

Due to earlier successes of the movement, the establishment of self-help alternatives and peer-support programs are ongoing in most areas of the country. Recently, movement efforts to influence policy have focused on two main areas. The first area of focus involves challenging the opposition's campaigns to impose forced treatment on psychiatric patients in the community (Involuntary Outpatient Commitment, Assertive Community Treatment). This also includes fighting efforts to change state laws to broaden commitment standards (making it easier to commit people to treatment against their will). The second area of focus includes the ongoing efforts to have and maintain a voice with influence in decision-making about policy at the national level.

### "No Forced Treatment"

Campaigns to fight introduction of outpatient commitment laws at the state level (such as Kendra's Law in New York State, passed after a young girl was pushed into the path of a subway train by a man who was mentally ill) have been an important area of contention for the movement. Outpatient commitment is a court order that requires a person to take medication on an outpatient basis; if compliance is not obtained, the person will be hospitalized or given the medication by force. In other words, you are sentenced to medication, and possibly to participation in outpatient treatment programs as well. Movement activists claim that sentencing to treatment is not acceptable, and that outpatient commitment is like being made a prisoner in your own home. Their slogan: "If it isn't voluntary, it isn't treatment" points out the fine line between treatment and punishment.

The movement by mental health advocacy groups like National Alliance for the Mentally Ill (NAMI) to promote such treatment laws demonstrates their differences with the c/s/x movement. NAMI (www.nami.org) has historically represented family members of psychiatrized persons who have lobbied to get more and earlier intervention for people in the community. They are currently campaigning to extend commitment laws beyond the current "harmful to self or others" designation and include "evidence of imminent deterioration" as grounds for involuntary commitment. The argument is made by NAMI lobbyists, particularly those of the Treatment Advocacy Center (www.psychlaws.org), that people who do not take their medication are likely to be dangerous, and therefore people should be forced to take medications for their own good, and the good of the community.

C/s/x movement activists make the counter-claim that rights are violated when people are sentenced to forced treatment when they have not committed a crime, but are viewed as being potential criminals. In the case of new experimental mental health courts and treatment "diversion" programs, the c/s/x movement takes the position that people should be punished for a crime they committed and not be "sentenced to treatment." They argue that no other category of patients (except those with tuberculosis) is forced to take treatment against their will. In addition, while arguing against a dangerousness supposition, they also point out that other categories of potentially dangerous people such as drinking drivers or even people who threaten spousal abuse are not punished before the fact, only after. C/s/x activists are, in turn, accused of encouraging the psychiatrized to "die with their rights on" by maintaining their right to avoid unwanted treatment.

This is a very contentious issue. In some states, such as California, the effort to introduce such bills has resulted in spirited public debate and demonstration. The outpatient commitment bill in California resulted in an upsurge of activity in the movement, as people have came together in response to this threat to civil liberties. Sally Zinman, executive director of the California Network of Mental Health Clients, described it this way: "We didn't even know about it [when the law was introduced]. But after that, we vowed that it would never happen again. We made a commitment to make sure that our people would be there to voice their opinions whenever and wherever this issue was brought to the table" (quoted in *The Key, NMHC-SHC Newsletter*: Vol. 6, No. 1, Spring 2000).

The first campaign was successful in defeating the bill; subsequently, its reintroduction in another legislative session was passed in spite of movement efforts.

These are excerpts from a May 2002, News Alert distributed by the SCI mailing list:

> June 12 is D Day for California clients. [We] have been campaigning for almost four years to defeat attempts in California to increase forced treatment. The attempt has metamorphosed into three shapes with 3 different bill numbers. It is now AB 1421 (Helen Thomson, Davis) and proposes an involuntary outpatient commitment program. . .

> The proponents of AB 1421 are waging a vigorous public relations
> campaign, exploiting the stereotype of the violent mental patient and
> increasing the public's fear of people with mental disabilities. . . Help us
> defeat this bill. Help us to defeat this attempt to turn back the clock on
> our rights and recovery. Write the Chair of the Health and Human
> Services Committee. In Support, Sally Zinman (SCI Internet bulletin
> "Rights under Siege" 5/23/02).

Such campaigns are shaped and limited by the context of the public view
of mental illness, as well as the power and resources of the opposition.
The current climate is not a healthy one for demanding rights for "the
mentally ill," because public sentiments have shifted away from these protections toward social control of deviant behaviors. Proponents of forced
treatment with biological psychiatry are gaining ground as outpatient
commitment laws are introduced in states around the country. This is addressed in the discussion of Goal 4, in which the opposition becomes a tar-
get of action.

## National Policy Representation

It is difficult to have a voice when your views are being discredited.
Nevertheless, movement activists have increasingly found a place at the
table in mental health policymaking. Recently Dan Fisher, M.D., a psychiatric survivor from the National Empowerment Center in Lawrence, Mass.,
was appointed to the President's New Freedom Commission for Mental
Health in June 2002. According to Ellen Barry writing for the Boston
Globe: "The yearlong commission, which has ten [fifteen] members, is
charged with studying America's mental health system and reporting back
on barriers to care, as well as successful models of community based care.
Also represented on the commission are numerous psychiatrists and a representative of the pharmaceutical company, Eli Lilly" (Barry 2002:C2).

Fisher was the only commissioner who had personally experienced
treatment by psychiatry or been active in a consumer/survivor group. This
was a coup for the movement. Although it was recognized to be another
token representation of the movement position in the midst of psychiatrists
and "Big Pharma," each opportunity must be taken and used as fully as possible. Lawyer-advocate Susan Stefan (2000) was also involved in the
Commission's report writing, and both representatives communicated actively with the movement about the process. In addition, open comment sessions were scheduled at every meeting, and the schedule was carefully
watched in order to have c/s/x activists available at every opportunity for

public comment. The Commission held its meetings at different cities around the country, and c/s/x presence was carefully coordinated in order to have the "rights and protection from abuse" position represented as well as the "need more treatment" position which is more commonly heard.

Movement activists are not naïve about these opportunities, even as they work to take advantage of them. As Judi Chamberlin noted (quoted in a "Support Coalition News Analysis" e-mail), "Back in 1979 President Carter also had a blue ribbon commission. There was only one token psychiatric survivor/mental health consumer on that commission, too. We're in the same position 23 years later" (6/19/02).

Meanwhile, the sole ex-patient Commissioner Dan Fisher was informed that the federal funding for his National Empowerment Center ($400,000 which was eighty percent of its yearly budget), as for all of the Technical Assistance Centers that had been promised funding, had been summarily cut by the federal government. An outraged campaign to protest the cuts with calls and letters proved to be effective, and the promised funds were restored; but then the funds were cut again (see chapter five).

Activists responded to the President's "New Freedom Commission" by creating an alternative "People's True Freedom Commission" including members from the c/s/x movement, the American Association of People with Disabilities and the ADA (Americans with Disabilities Act) Watch among others. The movement coalition arranged for a massive "freedom rally" demonstration and teach-in for the APA meetings in San Francisco on May 18, 2003.

## GOAL 4. TALKING BACK TO THE "MENTAL HEALTH MOVEMENT": "I AM NOT A CASE AND I DON'T NEED TO BE MANAGED!"

An important impetus for movement activities is the propensity of well-meaning citizens, professionals, corporations, and government officials to speak for people who have been psychiatrized. Conflicting views of what is necessary, helpful, and harmful are rampant. Historically, people who have been diagnosed and treated for mental illness have often been treated as voiceless and insignificant. When their voices are heard, they are disregarded in view of their madness. In today's world, some of the protagonists in the c/s/x battle for voice include National Alliance for the Mentally Ill (NAMI), the pharmaceutical industry ("Big Pharma") and the field of psychiatry itself.

As mentioned in chapter four, their perceived "lack of insight" gives activists instant discrediting if they disagree with the experts or the well-meaning community at large. At a larger level of public communication, this expert position is exploited to demean the efforts of the movement in general. In an effort to balance the insight gap, I will describe NAMI (National Alliance for the Mentally Ill) through the eyes of the c/s/x movement, as NAMI has historically had the upper hand in describing the troublesome radicals who resist treatment and undermine the power of psychiatry. The disputes between NAMI and the c/s/x movement will be described at length to reveal current issues, power struggles, and campaigns to maintain the power and credibility of voice as well as protect rights and the availability of choice and self-determination.

## Influencing the System

NAMI was formed in September, 1979 (Isaac & Armat 1990:265). It dates from the days when parents were blamed for their children's illness and closed out of the doctor-patient relationship for reasons of confidentiality. In an effort to improve treatment for their relatives, greater input in the process, and peace of mind for themselves, NAMI lobbied for change in the mental health system, and formed support groups to provide assistance, education, and coping skills for "family members" of people in the psychiatric system.

As the medical model or brain disease model of psychiatry has flourished, NAMI has heavily supported the research and development of these theories and treatments through lobbying for NIMH brain disease funding. NAMI has been quite successful in its efforts, has grown enormously, and has many chapters all around the U.S. It is also known to have an understandably symbiotic relationship with pharmaceutical companies, some of which provide significant funding for NAMI operations and activities, which in their turn promote the extensive use of medications and expansion of psychiatric treatment (Silverstein 1999).

Unlike the c/s/x movement, NAMI has is a very strong national organization and many local chapters which have more or less fidelity to the national mandates. Especially since it has become politically correct to do so, they have tried to include a segment of mental health consumers in their organization. This has caused much strife as consumers who "talk back" within their councils and boards have found their own voices and challenged some of the NAMI policies. However, there are plenty of docile consumers who are on display as "good" NAMI consumers (parallel to the "good patients" mentioned in chapter four). Meanwhile the "NAMI mommies," as they are sometimes derisively called, continue to work for more and better medications and easier routes to forced treatment.

*Competing Interests*

NAMI is known in the c/s/x movement for encouraging family members to lie about violent behavior in order to get their children committed, and even to use tactics like throwing around furniture to make things look worse than they really are—all for "the good" of their offspring who need help because they refuse to take their medication. According to Dr. E. Fuller Torrey, families do this because they "have no choice ... thus, ignoring the law, exaggerating symptoms, and outright lying by families to get care for those who need it are important reasons the mental illness system is not even worse than it is" (Torrey 1997a:152).

Exposure of these practices, such as alerts sent through the Internet, brings a moral victory over the enemy. Yet ordinary people who want control over "dangerous mental patients" see these NAMI tactics as understandable methods to get a person help under the circumstances. The rights of the psychiatrized are easily disregarded, even discarded, in the name of help. They are thus treated as less than human. This is why activists resist such practices, insisting that their human rights should be as undeniable as anyone else's. Why can their rights be so easily violated, they ask, when they have committed no crime?

Even activists who accept the medical model believe their rights should be protected. At the other end of the spectrum, there are psychiatrized individuals who have "good insight," having "internalized their oppression" enough to turn their rights over to someone else "when they get crazy". One psychiatrist I met who "is bipolar" takes this position in her own treatment plan. She calls herself a "prosumer" and claims to hold the wisdom of both sides of the argument.

Understandably, this psychiatrist is a heroic figure to the NAMI membership, and anathema to the c/s/x movement. To those in between, she is a concerned psychiatrist who has some insight into what it means to be mentally ill. Talking back to someone in her position is a challenge, and can be seen to represent a battle of "competing insights" in this very subjective experiential world of opposing views. It is the power to define the truth that makes the difference. Whose truth?

*Direct Confrontations*

A campaign carried out by Support Coalition brought ridicule and exposure to California's NAMI organization, which apparently glued together pages of its magazine, The JOURNAL, before distribution in order to censor an article by its editor. The headline of the internet news brief (NAMI Comes

Unglued) reported the details of this incident, including the censored text and a statement by its author, who was censored (and fired) for expressing a view that challenged the NAMI party line (*MindFreedom Journal* #44, 2001:27).

This exposure created turmoil in NAMI's ranks, as the censorship revealed a schism in the group and exposed a power play by the conservative side of the disagreement. These victories are invisible except to those who are involved, and yet they have great importance within the ranks of the movement and the other players in the field. Small power shifts and disagreements can carry great weight.

A central figure in the movement's pantheon of psychiatrists is E. Fuller Torrey, M.D. Torrey and his colleague, Mary Zdanowicz, are leaders of a group that is linked to NAMI, but became a separate organization because of its radical agenda. This organization, the Treatment Advocacy Center, has as its major purpose the promotion of Involuntary Outpatient Commitment laws in every state. Torrey and Zdanowicz's names appear in local papers around the country, headlining columns that promote local forced treatment ordinances by highlighting violent behavior by people with untreated mental illness. This is part of their media campaign. It depends on one's point of view whether this is seen as reasonable and warranted activity, or as despicable underhanded dishonesty and manipulation. The efforts of the c/s/x movement to highlight Torrey's activities and bring him shame have had mixed results, but efforts continue. Targeting Torrey in this way serves as a highly motivating campaign for many movement members and serves to build identity and strength in the movement.

Recently, Torrey's attitude of dismissive disdain toward c/s/x activism has become more of a direct attack on movement activities. This may be an indicator that the movement is becoming more effective and he is acknowledging it instead of ignoring it (that is, working against its goals without giving it recognition). In an early encounter, he published an essay in *Psychiatric Services* attacking the use of the word "survivor" by members of the movement: "Since the early 1980s a small number of consumers have identified themselves as 'psychiatric survivors,' but the term now appears to be becoming respectable, even politically correct. For example, the Center for Mental Health Services, a national model for political correctness, now uses the term 'consumers/survivors' in some of its publications" (Torrey 1997b:143).

Torrey goes on to say that by opposing psychiatry and involuntary hospitalization or medication, "psychiatric survivors and civil liberties lawyers have made it virtually impossible to treat such patients when they have no insight into their illness or their need for treatment. . . The policies espoused by 'psychiatric survivors' have thus led to a large number of non-survivors" (Torrey 1997b:143).

Movement activists responded with a call over the Internet for a barrage of letters-to-the-editor responses to his presumptuous attack. Apparently the number of responses received was record-breaking; no other article in the history of the journal had generated such a response. As the journal editor noted, "Many of the letters were from persons who identified themselves as psychiatric survivors and wrote to protest our publication of the commentary after reading an alert on the Internet by Support Coalition International, the publisher of *Dendron News*" (Mahler 1997:601). As a result, the editor created a special section devoted to this exchange, and excerpts from twenty of the seventy letters received were included as a rebuttal to Torrey's inflammatory piece.

Mahler's published letter begins, "In his Taking Issue commentary . . . Torrey . . . defamed several membership-based advocacy organizations. We help lead these organizations. In some instances, we were among their founders. We are all psychiatric survivors. Let us introduce ourselves . . ." (Mahler 1997:601). This is followed by brief quotes from Jay Mahler, Rae Unzicker, Janet Foner, David Oaks, and Judi Chamberlin, all long-term c/s/x activists, introducing themselves as "survivors" to the readers of *Psychiatric Services*.

In the same segment, Joseph Rogers' letter also appears, with this rebuttal quote:

> [Torrey] is wrong to blame the mental patients' rights movement-specifically those who call themselves 'survivors'—for the deaths of about half a million 'nonsurvivors' of mental illness. Yes, mental illness can kill you. But these deaths cannot be laid on the doorstep of those of us who oppose forced treatment. As a patients' rights activist, I am increasingly certain that the deaths of nonsurvivors have been caused by the failure to create an effective, comprehensive system of care. We need to work toward a system that provides early opportunities for help based on what people need and want" (Mahler 1997:602).

This series of events represents a victory of voice for the movement—and this time there was an audience, as this journal is widely read by psychiatrists and other mental health professionals.

Dr. Torrey has recently been joined by another "extremist psychiatrist" (a c/s/x label), Dr. Sally Satel, whose vituperative attacks on the movement and its supporters have received significant exposure. Satel's recent book, *P.C., M.D.: How Political Correctness is Corrupting Medicine* (2000) includes an entire chapter on the c/s/x movement entitled "Inmates Take Over the Asylum" in which she attacks both the movement and the government agencies (for example, the Center for Mental Health Services) that have supported it over the years with policies and funding. She calls for an end to funding of self-help and peer support programs, and to funding of the annual Alternatives conferences that have been so important to the movement. She uses an approach similar to Torrey's, opening the chapter with a horror story about a woman who commits suicide after being freed by a judge who "openly lamented the absence of any legal mechanism to make sure she received medical help" (2000:45).

Satel goes on to say:

> In fact, such a mechanism does exist. In a form of involuntary treatment called outpatient commitment, a court may order a regime of therapy and medication, and the patient may be rehospitalized if she fails to comply. Because of activism by a small but vocal group of former psychiatric patients, however, supported by civil liberties lawyers, thousands of people like Ray are not receiving the treatment they need to get well or at least to be safe. These activists call themselves "consumer-survivors" (also "psychiatric survivors") (Satel 2000:45).

Then she makes a point about the use of acceptable names for the movement:

> The term "consumer" denotes a user of mental health services, and "survivor" refers to one who has endured psychiatric care. "Survivor" is not used in this term in the same sense as "cancer survivor," someone who has had cancer and survived it, says the psychiatrist and researcher E. Fuller Torrey. "Rather," he points out, "it is being used like 'Holocaust survivor,' an individual who has been unjustly imprisoned and even tortured." [Here, Satel is quoting Torrey's position from the *Psychiatric Services* piece referred to above.] (Satel 2000:45-46).

Satel claims that the c/s/x movement wrongly obstructs the power of psychiatry:

> Some consumer-survivors have requested that the mental health profession "make an apology to consumers for past abuses of power" [quoted from a dialogue between consumers and psychiatric nurses sponsored by CMHS in Washington, D.C. 1999]. As we will see, radical consumer-survivors are the ones who more properly owe apologies to patients for standing in the way of constructive treatments and policies (Satel 2000:46).

She also touts the virtues of the NAMI organization and mentions the on-going debate:

"One of the voices against the anti-psychiatry extremism of consumer-survivors is the so-called family movement, led by the National Alliance for the Mentally Ill. . . Radical consumer-survivors can be counted on to reject virtually any good idea that NAMI favors" (2000:64-65).

The die is cast. In the rest of the chapter, Satel presents quotations from many c/s/x activists and leaders, quotes she has carefully mined and referenced from movement websites and published accounts. She uses them with obvious disdain, in a determined effort to undermine and discredit the movement using its own words. I find it fascinating that these psychiatric interlocutors can take the very language of the movement and use their expertise to undercut its credibility, in much the same way that this happens under psychiatric "treatment conditions" when acceptable discourse is defined by the dominant player. The two positions can exist in the same space; it is the reader's viewpoint that determines the interpretation.

The goal of Satel's book is to return medicine to a position of undisputed expertise by discrediting the various efforts to make it more responsive to the needs of groups (nurses, consumer-survivors, women, minorities, and others) who are challenging its authority and practice. "A clarion call," says reviewer Sherwin Nuland, M.D. He continues, "One after another, Satel takes on the central planks in the platform of PC [politically correct] medicine and replies to them with a devastating barrage of documentation, leavened by her own clinical and personal observations" (Satel, 2000: back cover).

The movement fought back. Activists discovered that Dr. Satel was being considered for an important post as a mental health consultant to the Bush administration, shortly after her attacks on the Center for Mental Health Services, the government agency that has provided support to the movement and to the development of self-help programs over the years, precisely because of CMHS support to the movement. Again, a barrage of e-mail was begun, this time to Charles Curie, the new director of SAMHSA (the Federal parent agency of CMHS). (Curie, interestingly enough, had been a staunch backer of peer support programs in Pennsylvania.) How could it be, people asked, that extremist Dr. Sally Satel is being considered for such a post?

Meanwhile, CMHS funding to exemplary consumer-survivor groups that existed as Technical Assistance Centers for self-help groups and peer support drop-in centers was suddenly cut. An Internet "News Update" from MindFreedom.org reported that:

a former top executive for Eli Lilly, a company that manufacturers psychiatric drugs, is the Bush official who is trying to immediately shut the doors of mental health consumer/psychiatric survivor national technical assistance centers. Action: Fax a civil message . . . While Daniels may be the one with the hand on the spigot, the ideologue who has publicly called for "overnight" termination of such funding is the latest advisor on mental health to Pres. Bush, Sally Satel. Satel works for the enormous corporate think tank, American Enterprise Institute (www.MindFreedom.org, 9/11/02).

The bulletin went on to point out that two board members of the American Enterprise Institute (with website listed) were drug company executives.

### An Ongoing Battle

Thus, the war goes on. The interests of psychiatry and the drug companies, along with NAMI and its involuntary-treatment activists, compete with the interests of individuals who have survived the mental health system and want to protect others from being harmed. It is a challenge to monitor, research, and respond to the activities of "the enemy" including developments in pharmacological research, human rights issues in research ethics, and positions presented in the media. Such battles are constantly being fought, requiring great energy and attention from activists and generally invisible to the public in their everyday life. They are battles of principle, competing interests, and influence.

There are many other areas of contention I have not covered in this chapter. Nearly every medical, legal, cultural, and marketing development relating to psychiatric treatment provides material for uncovering and debating the different interests and points of view. The small and large campaigns of the movement focus on maintaining its goal for representation, claiming voice in the conversations that will affect the lives of people who are diagnosed and treated by psychiatry. They focus on maintaining rights and protection from forced treatment in an era when the arguments for forced treatment are gaining ground.

Small power plays make a huge difference on this playing field, where the power of experts, interests of family members, and the experiential knowledge of psychiatric consumer/survivors are continually at odds. Often the battles become personalized, like the ongoing interactions between Oaks, Mahler, Satel and Torrey, as the alternative voices of c/s/x activists are pitted against the experts who use their professional authority to discredit the voices of the movement. The work of c/s/x activists is a continuing daily struggle to pursue the goals of the movement as well as maintain the advances of the movement's last thirty years.

Chapter Six
# The Politics of Identity, Power and Knowledge

## COMING TO TERMS WITH COMPLEXITY

The complexity of the consumer/survivor/ex-patient movement has made it a complicated topic for study. What seems simple on the surface ("oh, that anti-psychiatry movement" or "oh, that cult" or "oh, the consumer movement") reveals several layers of tension and contradictory positions. One of my earliest experiences in the field was in a conference group where radical ex-patients came together to share their experiences, and two participants revealed that they were taking medications. They were derided and discredited by the more radical participants in a way that reminded me of African-Americans being called Oreos or Jim Crow by their peers.

Later in the session, a parallel between the survivor stance and the natural childbirth movement also became evident. Participants made heroic claims about how much they had suffered at the hands of psychiatry, comparing stories just as I had heard mothers talk about their ability to suffer long hours of labor without succumbing to the offers of a spinal anesthesia or pain medication. Strength and weakness, suffering and survival, purity and compromise: these comparisons drive divisive claims about who the true movement activists really are. They cause pain and conflicted feelings among many members.

Cliques and factions were revealed through the fault lines of these claims; yet all were part of the larger movement at this meeting, and enthusiastic solidarity was evidenced in the larger group despite the underlying differences. What was the movement identity? Who were the authentic

activists and why did they alienate and harass each other? Learning movement history and issues of power and identity in relation to psychiatry
helped to make the issues more clear.

More moderate consumer activists often express discomfort about the
radical position. They claim that it harms their credibility and hinders their
negotiations with funders and policymakers who prefer to work with docile
and cooperative representatives of the mental health community. People
who are considered normal are more comfortable working with mental patients who are most like them, people they can count on not to get too demanding at meetings or unexpectedly raise a fuss. Yet even Dr. Torrey points
to the effective tactic of using a "lunatic fringe" (1988:373) to influence response to your group's demands.

When I encountered people who identified as consumers in the early
fieldwork, I sometimes felt that they had sold out or depended too much on
psychiatric medications for their well-being. I was identifying with the more
radical activists. Some people who were heavily medicated were referred to
as "zombies" by proudly medication-free activists. Yet the people on medications were an important part of the movement's growth and outreach activities. What did it mean to be a member of this movement? Who should I
talk to if I wanted to get the real story? Later I gained a greater appreciation
for the more grassroots activists, some of whom used medications, who
worked every day in their communities advocating for people in a bureau-
cratic and unresponsive system, far from the drama of movement leadership
and annual conference proceedings.

When I encountered family members who were active in NAMI and
the mental health movement, who wanted to "bust stigma" and spread the
word about mental illness and treatment, I got another sense of difference.
I heard them speak of their sons or daughters with the language of brain disease and low expectations, and I heard them discuss what was needed in
terms of treatment options. Many NAMI members wanted to make it easier to put their relatives in the hospital against their will, on the basis of imminent deterioration rather than actual dangerous. This earlier path to
involuntary commitment was considered more humane. Hearing their arguments and assumptions, I could see their rationales but I resisted their standpoint, which reflected their own point of view yet failed to take the views of
their "consumers" into account. The providers gave a similar message of
overvaluing their own knowledge at the expense of recipients of treatment
and their right to informed consent. In one conversation with a hospital psychiatrist, I was told, "If we tell them about the side effects, they won't take
their medicine. Then we would just have to get a court order."

Listening to the family members and the providers talk about the needs of consumer/survivors was an important lesson in voice and difference, and an important lesson about the movement. The radical and conservative members of the c/s/x movement were speaking in different voices, but they were speaking for themselves. The c/s/x activists were speaking from different corners of the same side, and they were brought together by their similarities just as they were divided by their differences. Their common goal of achieving voice for consumers and survivors and ex-patients, rather than being spoken for by others, ultimately trumps their competing views of the appropriate relations with psychiatry. They came together at the conferences and expressed both their similarities and differences, like squabbling siblings who had a common enemy.

This lesson remained with me as I encountered the c/s/x movement in its many forms. Its diverse members call themselves the consumer/survivor/ex-patient movement in a fundamental recognition of difference and common purpose. Why do they choose this cumbersome name? The underlying recognition of the right to have a voice *and* the right to be different is a basic tenet of the movement and, in my view, has allowed it to survive over this thirty-year span.

Recognition of difference and respect for dissent is at the core of the movement. Quite possibly it has also kept the movement from achieving some of its goals, which can become contradictory and prevent a cohesive approach. To achieve voice, it is necessary to be heard. If competing voices are making claims and interfering with each other, clarity will not be achieved and competition will create rivalries and enmity. And yet the conservative and radical factions have enlivened each other, as the conversation continues and no party line has evolved to obscure or override the differences; thus the movement continues to represent diverse views.

## IDENTITY AND DIFFERENCE

At the first Highlander Conference, twenty of the most radical movement activists in the U.S. came together for a strategy meeting. Paradoxically, in the interest of time and efficiency, the planners had created an agenda and had assigned participants to work groups that would be addressing particular issues together in a tight and highly organized schedule. The resulting power struggle was remarkable.

First, in an effort to respect the organizers, participants did not express their frustration directly, but the group was subdued and talked behind the scenes while trying to be cooperative. Soon the challenge emerged as people openly declared their discomfort with the schedule, the agenda,

and the group assignments. In a full-scale combination of consensus and rebellion, the plan was overturned and a new one created as everyone sat in
the meeting room, in the circle of Highlander's rocking chairs.

Even a directive to take turns speaking in order around the circle was
felt to be oppressive by one group member, and that last vestige of order was
abandoned. And yet this dissent was celebrated and recognized as the spirit
of the meeting, as the new plan emerged and was carried out over the next
days. This scene represents to me the spirit of the movement: not efficient
or organized, not easily led; full of authentic dissenters who are willing to
work together on their own terms for the good of the group. This is a truly
contradictory movement that gets in its own way by remaining true to its
goals of respecting difference by promoting voice and self-determination.

There have been long-term divisions, as described, though it is possible
that these rivalries drive the factions to work harder to achieve their competing goals as well as divide and divert their energies. The movement is anything
but complacent. What is remarkable is that its members do see themselves as
part of the movement—whether they say consumer movement, consumer/sur-
vivor movement, or c/s/x movement (which is ordinarily used in print but also
spoken). Challenges like those of E. Fuller Torrey have brought movement ri-
vals together to claim their identity as survivors (Mahler 1997), and recent
funding cuts that threaten the diverse organizational structures of the movement (technical assistance centers such as National Empowerment Center, the
National Mental Health Consumers' Self-Help Clearinghouse, Consumer
Organization & Networking Technical Assistance Center) have also brought
diverse factions together against a common threat.

In spite of its divisive history, the movement's claim to be a social
movement on a par with other rights movements appears valid. For most
people who self-identify as members of the movement, there is a common
identity of having been psychiatrized, and this identity has a group awareness and common grievances. There is a shared grievance of loss of power,
stigmatization and injustice in the achieved master status of mental patient.
There is a shared experience of discrediting and betrayal of trust in the relationship defined by that status (revealed in the survivor narrative), and a
common goal of claiming the same rights as others in spite of the label of
psychiatric diagnosis. The use of peer-support self-help groups as a strategy
both for organizing and empowerment has provided an underlying unity, a
source of legitimization and also the experience of co-optation by the mental health system.

From the early days through its subsequent adaptations and elaborations (as described in chapter three), the movement has shown a diversity

that might be expected in a social movement that includes a variety of members, a goal of empowerment, and a loose organization without central control. The women's movement and the civil rights movement, for instance, have had various factions and divisive splits over the years. Claiming voice is itself a contentious process. When there is no central authoritative voice that claims to represent or dictate to a membership, the maturation process of the movement leads to different voices taking shape and claiming their right to speak, changing (and challenging) the movement over time. I believe this process characterizes the c/s/x movement's particular emphasis on claims to voice in tandem with claims to self-determination.

This is why the so-called language wars (both inside and outside the movement) are so important. The persistent debate over the right to decide what words to use in defining one's identity (as a movement, as an individual in the movement, and as an individual in relation to psychiatry) is a critical and ongoing aspect of the movement at both personal and collective levels. Claims to individual and collective power over definitions of self and identity are paramount in the assertion of the right to voice. Who has the right to speak? Who has the right to define? These themes are apparent in the movement itself as well as in its areas of contention with psychiatric authority.

The narratives that drive the movement place it in competition with the authoritative narratives of psychiatry. Uppity mental patients have been put in their place over and over again, yet they keep talking back. And the movement appears to be growing stronger. This is evidenced, as I have tried to demonstrate, by its increasingly visible presence in the media, in the national policy debates, and in various state campaigns regarding forced-treatment legislation. They are not running things, but they have a voice, and their presence is now mandated. Strong individual presence at many locations helps to keep the movement positions being heard. These individuals keep in touch with each other for strength and strategic support. The strength of movement presence in CMHS and the mental health system (self-help programs, increased inclusion of consumer voices at the levels of planning, service delivery, quality assurance, and outcomes measurement) has reached the point where psychiatrists like Torrey and Satel are attacking the movement directly, as well as CMHS itself for harboring such activists and giving them mainstream influence.

To claim voice and authority at the individual level, in relation to one's caretakers, takes personal strength, ingenuity, and a deep sense of the rightness of the self in the face of difference. It can be dangerous because the discourse of definition does not belong to the "patients" but to psychiatry. To beg to differ is to put oneself at risk, as such difference invites correction, which may indeed be provided against your will (and for your own good). Acceptance of psychiatric assistance invites one form of social control; refusal invites another. People in the movement have choices about what to accept, and can claim rightness in the face of opposition from other movement members as well.

## CHALLENGING THE DISCOURSE

To claim voice and authority in a collective sense, to talk back to psychiatry and its narrative in the larger realm, takes persistence, audacity and creativity far beyond that required at the individual level. At the collective level, personal risk is reduced. The players have gone beyond the confines of the help-seeking (private or public) setting, bringing the conversation into the public realm. Over the years, the mental health system has made accommodations in response to movement demands and claims, with efforts to include consumer voices at the table to make mental health reforms. The more conservative activists find this slow progress promising and acceptable, and want to continue good relations with their mentors.

Yet the more radical side continues to make competing claims by challenging the authority of psychiatry, the claims of the pharmaceutical industry, and their combined practices of expansion and control. For some activists, it is not enough to sit at the table. They want to change the table, or destroy the table and use another one altogether. Most recently, there were plans for a hunger strike protest in summer 2003 to call public attention to the lack of honesty in the knowledge claims and practices of psychiatry and the pharmaceutical companies. One challenge, among others, was for the psychiatric profession to offer proof of the biomedical model of mental illness. In a clash of competing knowledges and claims to authority, both sides claimed success and public attention was drawn to the issues. Dedicated activists will continue to develop such plans, and many others, in their effort to gain public recognition for movement voices and to challenge the oppressive authority of psychiatry.

In the continuing debate that represents the movement's challenge to the psychiatric discourse, there is a parallel between the private and the public experience. The practices of social control used against discreditable and discredited individuals are enlarged into practices that silence, disregard or discredit dissenting voices in the public arena. One way to discredit the movement itself is to discredit its members, and to discredit its supporters as well. Whether through action or non-action, the efforts of members of the psychiatric establishment to ignore, undermine or control the movement's persistent challenges to psychiatric authority display a patronizing certainty (as in, we are the experts, and we say these people and their supporters are wrong; not only wrong, but misguided, foolish, and in fact downright harmful) that is grounded by the cultural authority of the psychiatric narrative.

The recent change from total dismissal to active attack may reflect a growing competitive strength of the movement narrative, as it gains a place (however token) at the higher-level tables of policymaking and finds its way into the popular press as well. However, when claims made by c/s/x activists attempt to challenge psychiatric authority in its own domain, as with campaigns against electroshock, they sometimes fall on hard ground. With psychiatry's increased claims to expert knowledge through brain science and pharmaceuticals, directly challenging psychiatric authority on the public level, even with professional allies, is less culturally acceptable than it was in 1978. Yet the efforts will continue.

At the same time, the growth of the movement has put individual activists in a stronger position in relation to their service providers. Increased representation of consumer views in the mental health system brings more credibility to the competing discourse of the movement. These separate strands of movement effort intertwine and have seen varied results over time, in response to opportunities and challenges in the context of changing circumstances.

At a personal level, each conversation informed by knowledge of advocacy provides an opportunity for increased self-determination. As active patients or consumers find voice to express their needs and dissatisfactions, whether in doctor-patient relations or in newly-enhanced managed care grievance procedures, they are maintaining their right to speak and disagree. The growth of advocacy, in effect, undermines psychiatric hegemony one conversation at a time. Small victories in private exchanges may or may not change the psychiatrist, but can greatly change the recipient's experience of treatment and the self, as well as the quality of life when more choices are available. Collective awareness and encouragement of these interpersonal challenges provide strength and solidarity for ongoing activism.

## BEYOND THE MENTAL PATIENT IDENTITY

The consumer/survivor/ex-patient movement has reached some of its goals in enhancing the voice of the psychiatrized over the past thirty years. At the private level, opportunities to speak and rights protection have both increased. Non-treatment spaces like drop-in centers provide sites for advocacy and open peer-to-peer conversation. At the public level, the credibility of the consumer/survivor position has also increased, enlarging the choices and the collective authority of this opposing view. However, as with any movement, gains may be lost. Competing claims for resources, and for authority, make the continuation of these achievements a challenge and will affect the future of the movement. As we have seen, the opposition has recently succeeded in reducing government funds for c/s/x activities. Such external challenges have already increased movement strength by bringing rival leaders into alliance, enhancing their commitment and resolve. Given the history of the movement, the ongoing strength of this alliance is unpredictable.

A similar process of resistant identity development can be recognized at both private and public levels. This is the assertion of an alternative way to perceive and define experience, even if that way of perceiving has been discredited by psychiatry and by the public at large, and even if it has been defined as mental illness. The experience of becoming a mental patient (Scheff 1999) appears to have been transformed in the c/s/x movement experience. Claiming voice and authority, expressing one's personal experience and one's experience of psychiatry, is an assertion of the self at both individual and collective levels. It is a rejection of the power of existing authority, professional or social, to define the self. In the movement, this assertion can become a celebration of deviant identity and collective experience, as well as a claim to be recognized as a human being.

## A DIFFERENT KIND OF IDENTITY POLITICS

This reclamation process is a form of identity politics, yet I believe it is a different form from that proposed by Anspach (1979). The competing narratives, the "self against science" experience, are occurring at both personal and collective levels. Going beyond a celebration of one's deviant identity and challenging the public's view of it (as in early "mad liberation" days), there is a simultaneous challenge to the right of others to bestow the deviant identity itself.

For instance, if someone identifies as gay or lesbian, or as female, or as Arab-American or African-American, these are identity realities that may be seen as internal to or owned by that person. Then it is the negative perception of the identity as socially discrediting that is challenged by the identity movements of these rights groups. We are this, yes, and we are proud to be who we are. Control of definition, or the right to define the value and meaning of an identity, is an important aspect of identity politics. Stigmatized groups may celebrate their identities and resist the stereotypes and discrimination of others' views of who they are, while working to re-frame their identity and change society's response into a more positive one.

In the c/s/x movement, I believe there is a difference. The mental pa-tient identity is an achieved identity status, officially assigned to a person by an expert other, confirmed by societal response. Whether it is considered an internalized response to societal reaction (a label), as described by Scheff (1999), or a biological condition diagnosed by psychiatry, it is a way of framing reality based on a person's troublesome and different behaviors and thoughts. The person is labeled, medicalized, psychiatrized—then experi-ences the consequences of this new identity status (whether experienced as beneficial or harmful).

The discredited identities of the other movements mentioned above are deviant ascribed identities. These identities, through the process of iden-tity politics, are accepted, claimed, and redefined by their social movements. The c/s/x movement takes a more complex position that requires differenti-ating the internal and external identity attributions. The message is some-thing like this: (1) The identity that has been assigned to us, this label of psychiatric diagnosis, is harmful and disqualifying. (2) The treatments that result from the label are also harmful and dangerous. (3) By assigning the label, thus indicating the treatments, harm is being done.

In the case of mental illness, the label itself actually gives others the right to intervene in a person's life. In choosing its identity politics, the c/s/x movement has a choice: (1) reject the label by disqualifying the labelers' ex-pertise, thus avoiding the harm; (2) reject the linkage of the label with the harm, by promoting the development of other treatments; (3) claim the identity (madness) and celebrate it with mad pride, working to reclaim the meaning and redefine it for others in society; or, (4) accept the expertise be-hind the label, fight the stigma it entails, and welcome the treatments that approximate one's normalization.

The complexity of the consumer/survivor/ex-patient movement de-rives from the complexity of its identity politics. In the early mad liberation days, it came close to approximating the identity politics of claiming, re-defining and celebrating deviant identity. In the later movement, this highly politicized survivor/ex-patient position had to compete with the more re-formist consumer activities of the movement, resulting in the split over fed-eral funding and co-optation. In reality, as I have tried to demonstrate, the movement has included a range of responses to the labeling and the treat-ment, and particularly to the discrediting and the offenses to basic human rights such as forced treatment.

These complexities play out in the variety of identity politics. Some activists described in chapter four, who accept the medicalization and the diagnosis, are nonetheless resisting the totalizing identity of their psychiatric label and maintaining their right to negotiate for power and recognition in the defining/treating relationship. More radical activists, who reject both the diagnosis and the knowledge behind it, resist the right of psychiatry to define them and to determine what they need. And they publicly celebrate Mad Pride Day on July 14th, Bastille Day, chosen because some of the prisoners released were mental patients. This celebration of identity is used to build solidarity and pride in the movement, and to expose the issues to public view with parades and picket signs calling attention to psychiatric abuse and forced treatment as well as claiming mad pride.

C/s/x activists are resisting (1) the attribution, and (2) the power the attribution gives others over their lives. They are resisting the label, I believe, precisely because inherent in the label (and the labeling) is a disempowerment and discrediting that are not only stigmatizing, but also remove the right to self-determination. The stigma and discrediting are, of course, interpersonal, assigned or negotiated within all social relations, and especially in the defining relationship itself.

The psychiatric doctor-patient relationship assigns the stigmatizing label to one member of the dyad, and also gives the labeling member the power to define the other, which implies power over the other. To reject the label, or even just the meaning of the label, is to challenge this power and thus to invite invalidation and social control. The power relations are imbalanced in a significant way, and this imbalance is both socially sanctioned and legally enhanced.

## A RADICAL COMPARISON

To gain a fuller understanding of this relation, a comparison to the African-American experience may be appropriate. As stated in chapter three, this sort of radical comparison (i.e., holocaust victims, experimental subjects, colonization), is an approach that often annoys and alienates allies of the movement. Yet activists often make these radical comparisons, to express their strong and resonant connection with other forms of human rights abuse and oppression. I will make such a comparison here in an effort to elaborate the experience of psychiatrization to further extend the analysis.

In the master-slave relation, the master (as a member of a social group, which has defined the norms and values of the situation) defines what it is to be a slave, and defines the rules of the relationship. The slaves are likely to have their own definitions of what it is to be a slave, but the master's definition is the authorized version. Rule-breaking by the slave leads to punishment. Rule-breaking by the master might bring negative sanctions, but given the power relations, it would be the master's prerogative and most likely to the master's benefit. (Since the master has the power to make the choice, this is a reasonable assumption when such a choice is made. For instance, if the choice is to bring the slave in for a nice dinner, it will perhaps make the master feel benevolent; even if the master's peers negatively sanction the rule-breaking behavior, there must be some perceived benefit that makes the action desirable as a way to exercise power). If the rules are broken, whether for humanitarian purposes or for punishment and control, the choice is still the master's.

If the slaves break the rules, they will be punished, unless they do it behind the scenes (with hidden transcripts). They are challenging the reality in which the relationship is defined; more importantly, they are challenging the right to define it. Even slaves who wished to escape were labeled with psychiatric illness (drapetomania) which redefined their reality (desiring freedom) as madness.

The civil rights movement, in which black men and women fought for equality (supported by their allies), involved a claim to the right to decide what it meant to be black. Being black was no longer to be "a slave," though attitudes and practices were still discriminatory. The civil rights laws went further to define discrimination on the basis of color as unacceptable, in an effort to transform cultural norms and practices to a more desirable social standard.

In the identity politics of the civil rights movement, the claim was made that "being black" was "no worse" than being white, that equal treatment was required; just as "being gay" is not a basis for discrimination by straights, and "being female" is not defined as being less than male. In fact, being black was beautiful, and other celebrants claimed their own identity statuses. In identity politics, the claims can move from "worse (discredited)" to "no worse (equal)" to "even better (celebration)." So, how does this relate to identity politics of the c/s/x movement?

In comparison, I want to make the point that being "mad" (except in the early days of the movement) is not a parallel experience. To c/s/x movement activists the logic might look like this: If "being black" still meant "being a slave" with the power differential that entails, then "being a mental patient" and "being black" would be parallel. "Being a mental patient" is not an identity for which a radical position leads to a claim that "being a mental patient is beautiful," because the identity is not an internal one that can be reclaimed from others; it is an external one that defines a person in terms of power relations as in the slavery analogy. According to the c/s/x movement, it is an oppressive identity that is achieved through its assignment by others, precisely because of one's difference or madness (as described by Scheff's [1999] labeling process). The very difference that is being celebrated, then, in "mad pride" is essentially the difference that is one's identity before being labeled, and, in effect, after rejecting the label through resistance of psychiatric authority. This would allow celebration of the ascribed aspects of one's own unusual identity or difference that attracted the attention of psychiatry in the first place.

## MAD PRIDE?

These are equality movements, demanding recognition of status and identity. In the early days of the c/s/x movement, "mad liberation" was an important slogan that called for freedom and voice for people who had been incarcerated in mental institutions, with damaging treatments and no rights protection. It called for equal rights for mental patients. It also celebrated the mad identity, its freedom and spontaneity, in a natural fit for the era of the early 1970s. This is a different era; society and the mad movement have evolved from the days of the electric Kool-Aid acid test to Internet action alerts about human rights abuses.

There is an ongoing Mad Pride aspect to the c/s/x movement, and I believe it is celebrated today in a different sense. Mad Pride actions celebrate the right to voice, and they call attention to psychiatric abuse, as well as commemorating the history of the movement, its continuity, and its energy. They celebrate a pride in the movement, with all its names and labels. There are not any good names for this movement; there are too many good names for the movement. None of them describe it exactly, and no one knows that better than its members.

In fact, the more reformist movement members who make claims about destigmatizing their mental illness do not celebrate Mad Pride Day. Ironically, it seems that the parallel to the equal rights and stigma-busting identity-politics position of other movements may be reflected most strongly in the claims of those who challenge the c/s/x movement, not those who support it. The identity politics that approximate the "mental illness is beautiful" model represent, instead, the position of the other mental health movement (including the NAMI counter-movement) that supports the biomedical brain disease model of mental illness, and claims to represent the interests of the mentally ill. These are the people who discredit most c/s/x activists (even the reformist ones) as too radical, and, as I have explained, lobby for legislation to limit the rights of the mentally ill so that they can be treated against their will, for their own good. Thus the parallel to identity politics in other rights movements, which seems as though it would be so direct (Mad Pride), is seen to be somehow skewed ("Destigmatize Mental Illness") because it maintains the oppressed position described above.

And so there is another irony. While the c/s/x movement is working hard to be inclusive, and represent a range of persons who are oppressed by psychiatry, the consumers who take the arch-conservative mental health movement position described above (analytically, a fully-internalized deviance, medicalized deviance, fully-psychiatrized position) are seen by the more radical activists to represent the very most oppressed psychiatrized group. They are seen in fact to represent the experience of false consciousness, accepting their psychiatric oppression, yet the c/s/x movement is still fighting for their rights. They could be seen as a part of the larger movement, representing the most conservative consumer position. They tend to be the most acceptable (and celebrated) by mental health professionals and family members (as long as they know their place) and thus the most visible consumers, giving the perception that they in fact are the mental health consumer movement. As we have seen, there is more to the movement than that.

To continue the analysis, this conservative stigma-busting group of mentally ill people would probably include those who successfully internalized their deviance (in the Scheff sense) and accepted their medical patient (brain disease) identity. An example described earlier is the psychiatrist who identifies as bipolar and claims her right to equality, yet planfully (through a legal advance directive) gives up her control to others when she becomes ill. This position can be translated as the normalizing position offered by Anspach (1979), represented as follows: Yes, I have a brain disease, and I want the right to be treated like other people, as long as I try to be normal (though I am less than you normals, so please help me and others like me when we lose control, when we are wrong and claim not to be ill or refuse help).

The c/s/x movement considers this situation a sad case of false consciousness and internalized oppression (she even became a psychiatrist) which is actually harmful to the movement. There is a fine line between the weakest link and the enemy, and this doctor may represent that point. Yet she is still seen as being oppressed by psychiatry.

This conservative activist position can be seen as a form of identity politics, claiming equality for the mentally ill (such as parity of insurance for psychiatric care, including forced treatment), even celebrating the identity with support groups (such as NDMDA) and going public with the diagnosis to fight stigma. But, at the same time, this position is based on the discrediting and dehumanizing claim that the mentally ill are equal with others only when they are normalized, when they are receiving treatment, when they have good insight into their illness. And this allows those with false consciousness to work to further oppress their mentally ill peers, by taking the position that their deviance requires intervention to allow them to become not-quite-normal once again, and supporting forced treatment interventions in the community for their own good. This "qualified rights" position looks like a rights position, but actually maintains the status quo and promotes oppression. (It's like saying that blacks, women, gays and lesbians are equal, but only as long as they stay in their place.) In other words, they want voice, and they want choice—but they don't trust themselves to make the right choices because they are mentally ill.

## THE RADICAL STANCE

The inclusion of the ultra-conservative group in the c/s/x movement may be far-fetched, as it is a stretch to the far right of consumer on the activist continuum. Yet it serves as a useful contrast for analysis. In a sense, the question becomes whether they are speaking in their own voices, or simply the voice of their psychiatrized false consciousness.

In comparison, the rest of the movement takes a more radical stance. From this radical position, one might see the situation of being a slave (in relation to master), rather than being black (in relation to white), as a parallel to being psychiatrized (as a patient in relation to psychiatrist): a situation in which one's very being is defined by others (others who exist in a socially defined and defining relation to you, their status to your status) who have the right and the power to make and apply the rules on their own terms. And, they do it with the support of a social system that approves of their practice and gives them the power. Disagreeing with them, presenting your own point of view, is to be by definition wrong, and perhaps even taken as a sign of worsening illness. Challenging their authority is deviance and requires treatment, or defiance and requires correction and discipline. Efforts to redefine the relationship will require being put in one's place.

My description here is unconventional in an effort to experientially convey the differential logic of viewing the situation from the psychiatrized point of view. It is more possible to understand the ironies of the c/s/x position if one is able to see it, to take the position if only for a moment. Otherwise the view of the dominant narrative maintains its position and the alternative claim has little credibility except as an anomaly, or an uppity and irrational patient. This is where the voice of the movement needs to become partially present in the voice of analysis, without losing an analytic perspective.

The claim to a voice (diverse voices) is necessary in order for larger claims to gain credence. When the voice is discredited from the beginning, claims are easily dismissed if they are heard at all. The identity politics of the c/s/x movement relate less to the positive or negative definition of their identity, than to the right of others to define their identity in the first place, and then to further limit their credibility with the assumptions contained in the definition and in the defining relationship itself. Here lies the challenge to the expert knowledge that has created (and lives by) the diagnostic identities, as well as the corollary assumptions that define the realities of those who are diagnosed. It is an ultimate politics of identity, where they are demanding the power to be a part of the identity discussion. Otherwise, their deeply discredited identity leaves them voiceless, and useless except as objects of treatment and control: a potential source of profit by practitioners and the pharmaceutical industry.

It would be interesting to compare this movement with the successful attainment of voice in HIV/AIDS activism, and feminist trauma survivor groups as well. While these three groups share the acquisition of achieved identity in defining their status, the comparison of medical versus psychiatric conditions, the demand for making treatment more available versus rebelling against it, and the public response to their deviant status, make their experiences quite different while sharing many similarities. Untangling these complexities with further comparative exploration, as well as elaboration of the cultural and emotional impetus behind such complex social movements, will add new insights to the social movement literature.

## SCHEFF REVISITED

Revisiting Scheff (1999), we see that by resisting the sick role, the movement activists are asserting the right to define (to a greater or lesser degree) their own identity. Their rejection of the internalized deviant identity (assigned to them by societal reaction, as defined by Scheff) implies a position of power in the relationship that is not provided in Scheff's theory. They are moving beyond the "secondary deviance" definition in an attempt to define their own positions.

Scheff writes of the labeling process as a matter of rule breaking and deviance, followed by "negotiating a shared definition" (1999:123). This negotiation involves an imbalance of power (1999:128) that gives psychiatry "control over the definition of the situation" (1999:129) resulting in the psychiatrization of the individual and his or her identity. From then on, the identity exists, and the person exists, in relation to the psychiatrist and to the society that, in its reaction to deviance, has led the person to be psychiatrized: "The professional interrogator . . . can maintain control if the client cedes control to him because of his authority as an expert, because of his manipulative skill in the transaction, or merely because the interrogator controls access to something the client wants [treatment? freedom?]" (1999:129).

Scheff's description provides the labeled person little opportunity for agency in this interaction, other than the choice to cede control. It is surprising that the recent (1999) edition of his book does not include any mention of c/s/x activism. He does cite recent work by Breggin and Cohen (two of the movement's strongest professional allies) to support his points about the inadequacies of the biopsychiatric model. It is puzzling that the c/s/x movement itself, and consideration of personal agency and choice in the labeling process, are fundamentally ignored.

I propose to take Scheff's account one step further to recognize the active role of the patient, individually and collectively, in moving beyond passive patienthood and engaging the authority of psychiatry. By resisting the standard power differential, c/s/x activists are actively challenging, and perhaps changing, the terms of negotiation in the relationship. This self-versus-science or person-versus-psychiatry stance is enacted in the private and the public worlds, as noted above.

## THE POWER OF SMALL RESISTANCE

The continuum of activism begins in the doctor-patient relationship. Simple acts of resistance include issues of medication compliance, negotiation of treatment plans, and preparation of psychiatric advance directives. There is also a basic level of resistance to being identified by the label, exemplified by the following encounter.

An advocate with a longstanding diagnosis of bipolar illness, good medication compliance and insight into her illness, had a change in insurance coverage and was required to choose a new psychiatrist. Their first meeting was described to me as follows:

Advocate: Walks in and sits down.

Psychiatrist (looking through folder, not at patient): "Hmmm, let's see, okay, you're bipolar."

Advocate: "No, I'm [my name]."

This simple act of resistance exemplifies my research participants' underlying dissatisfaction with the way in which the power of psychiatry is exercised. An innocent triplet of conversational exchange, it was an immensely important moment in this advocate's life and was described to me with incredulous fury and fiery pride, exemplifying the emotional response to perceived abuse of psychiatric power which is a driving force behind the c/s/x movement and so hard for outsiders to understand.

To summarize, this power has the potential to dehumanize and deeply discredit the individuals who move into its circle of discourse. Once there, it is difficult to maintain one's self-worth and individual identity. Attempting to leave can result in the mobilization of more power against potentially "inappropriate" choices one might make outside the circle. An effort to remain as an active patient requires compromise and negotiation, as treatment compliance has consequences for daily life (short and long-term side-effects, stigma and discrimination, limitations on life choices). Non-compliance can result in more serious consequences.

## SPEAKING VOICE AGAINST POWER

Talking back to psychiatry occurs at all levels. It is rarely heard outside its immediate vicinity. Identity politics, the politics of identity in this case, is a constant negotiation of voice against power. The power to define oneself, or one's collectivity (as in gay and lesbian activism, black activism, women's activism) and to fight the associated stigma has different features when the label and its limitations have been assigned to you by others.

Moving the negotiation from the private to the public realm, dissenting voices are heard on different levels. At the local systems level there is increased representation in the mental health bureaucracy and in the managed care "consumer" feedback loop. These voices must compete with the authority claims of professionals and other advocacy groups who also claim to represent their interests. As evidenced in chapter five, those who define the discourse have a distinct advantage in discrediting the voices that challenge their position in the debate.

Negotiating for voice outside the mental health system is a more recent effort, enhanced by efforts to collaborate with other rights groups. Fighting against forced treatment and for basic rights has brought c/s/x activists into alignment with disability rights activists. Efforts to align with other rights groups have been challenging, partly because of the stigma of psychiatric diagnosis and the difficulty of identifying shared issues. Going beyond the identity politics of mental illness or mad liberation to issues of basic human rights and freedoms is an ongoing effort.

There is a core message in the c/s/x movement that society's current response to difference, with psychiatric labeling, forced treatment, and dehumanization is an affront to human rights. The core survivor narrative described in chapter four is a unifying framework that builds collective identity and purpose among individuals who have a variety of concerns and points of view. The challenge of gaining support from the general public and of joining with other movements is of strategic importance for the future of this movement. The everyday realities of its members are driven by their own internal identities as activists who resist the power of psychiatry to define their lives, in the various ways they choose to do their advocacy work. The movement will continue, as it has for thirty years, shaped by their choices, their alliances, and the response of psychiatry, the policymakers, and the public.

# Appendix A
# Conferences Attended

I. National Conferences Sponsored by Consumer/Survivor/Ex-Patient Movement

Alternatives '96: Creating Healing Alternatives for Real Health Care Reform. December 14–18, 1996. Orlando, FL

NARPA '97 Conference, National Association for Rights Protection and Advocacy. October 15–18, 1997. Daytona Beach, FL

Alternatives '98: Taking Charge Together. February 12–15, 1998. Long Beach, CA

NARPA '98 Conference, National Association for Rights Protection and Advocacy. November 19–22, 1998. Albany, NY

National Summit of Mental Health Consumers and Survivors. August 25–29, 1999. Portland, OR

Support Coalition Highlander Strategy Conference. March 23–26, 2000. Highlander Research and Education Center, TN

MIND AID: Decade of the Brain, Millennium of the Person Conference. May 30–31, 2000. New York, NY,

Alternatives 2000: A New Vision of Recovery. October 11–14, 2000. Nashville, TN

Support Coalition Highlander 2001 Strategy Planning Conference. March 22–25, 2001. Highlander Research and Education Center, TN

II. Statewide and Regional Conferences

Ninth Annual Pennsylvania Statewide Consumer Conference: Choices: Building Bridges to Alternatives. June 2–4, 1997. Erie, PA

Tenth Annual Pennsylvania Statewide Consumer Conference: Recovery: Body, Mind & Spirit. June 11–13, 1998. Philadelphia, PA

Allegheny County Consumer Support Program Conference: Choosing to Reach Your Dreams. October 9–10, 1998.

United Mental Health "We are Not Alone XIV" Conference. May 1, 1999. Pittsburgh, PA

Eleventh Annual Pennsylvania Statewide Consumer Conference: Celebrating Diversity, Supporting One Another. June 17–19, 1999. Pittsburgh, PA

Twelfth Annual Pennsylvania Statewide Consumer Conference: Embracing
Empowerment. June 7–10, 2000. Harrisburg, PA

Thirteenth Annual Pennsylvania Statewide Consumer Conference: Rights,
Dignity, Respect. May 22–25, 2001. Pocono Manor, PA

## III. National Mental Health Research Conferences (Sponsored by National Association of State Mental Health Program Directors National Research Institute, NASMHPD-NRI)

1998 NASMHPD-NRI 8th Annual Conference on State Mental Health
Agency Services Research, Program Evaluation and Policy: "Thinking
Outside the Box: Ethical Challenges in Public Mental Health Services
Research." February 1–3, 1998. Orlando, FL

1999 NASMHPD-NRI 9th Annual Conference on State Mental Health
Agency Services Research, Program Evaluation, and Policy: Uses of
Research, Outcome Assessment and Evaluation Findings for Multiple
Purposes." February 7–9, 1999. Alexandria, VA

Appendix B
# Websites

I. Sites of Consumer/Survivor/Ex-Patient Movement and Allies
    Adbusters MADPRIDE issue: www.prozacspotlight.org/madpride
    Alaska Mental Health Consumer Web: http://akmhcweb.org
    Alliance for Human Research Protection: www.researchprotection.org
    American Association of People with Disabilities: www.aapd-dc.org
    Antipsychiatry Coalition: www.antipsychiatry.org
    Bazelon Center for Mental Health Law: www.bazelon.org
    California Association of Mental Health Patients' Rights Advocates:
        www. camhpra.org
    California Network of Mental Health Clients: www.cnmhc.org
    Consumer Organization & Networking Technical Assistance Center:
        www. contac.org
    Dr. John Breeding: www.wildestcolts.com
    Dr. Loren Mosher: www.moshersoteria.com
    Dr. Peter Breggin (ICSPP): www.breggin.com
    Dr. Thomas Szasz: www.szasz.com
    ECT.org: www.ect.org
    Grohol: www.grohol.com
    "Intentional Care" Initiative: www.intentionalcare.org
    Institute for the Study of Human Resilience: www.bu.edu/resilience
    Justice for All: www.jfanow.org
    Law Project for Psychiatric Rights: http://psychrights.org
    Lunatics' Liberation Front: www.walnet.org/llf
    MadNation: www.madnation.cc
    Madness (People Who): www.peoplewho.org
    Mental Disability Rights International: www.mdri.org
    Mental Health Alliance (UK): www.mind.org.uk/take_action/mha.asp
    Mouth Magazine: www.mouthmag.com
    National Association for Rights Protection & Advocacy:
        www.narpa.com
    National Conference on Organized Resistance: www.organizedresistance.org
    National Council on Disability: www.ncd.gov

National Empowerment Center: www.power2u.org
National Mental Health Consumers' Self-Help Clearinghouse:
    www.mhselfhelp.org
NO Force UK Campaign: http://pages.zdnet.com/cullyd/thenoforcecampaign
Pennsylvania Mental Health Consumer Association: www.pmhca.org
People Against Coercive Treatment (PACT): www.tao.ca/~pact
Psychiatrized.org: www.psychiatrized.org
The Rose Garden Children's Foundation: www.geocities.com/Stnektarios
Safe Harbor Project: www.AlternativeMentalHealth.com
Schizophrenia Drug-free Crisis Centre: www.jungcircle.com/Schizophrenia.html
State Hospital Cemetery Restoration Project: http://dsmc.info
Stop Shrinks: www.stopshrinks.org
Support Coalition International: www.mindfreedom.org
Survivors' Art Foundation: www.survivorsartfoundation.org
World Network of Users and Survivors of Psychiatry: www.wnusp.org
Zuzu's Place—Cooperative Living for Psychiatric Survivors:
    www.zuzusplace.org

## II. Related Sites

American Psychiatric Association: www.psych.org
American Psychological Association: www.apa.org
Center for Mental Health Services: www.mentalhealth.org
Center for Psychiatric Rehabilitation: www.bu.edu/cpr
Center for Reintegration: www.reintegration.com (sponsored by Eli Lilly)
International Association of Psychosocial Rehabilitation Services:
    www.iapsrs.org
Knowledge Exchange Network: www.mentalhealth.com
MIND (UK): www.mind.org
Missouri Institute of Mental Health Program in Consumer Studies & Training:
    www.cstprogram.org
National Alliance for the Mentally Ill: www.nami.org
NAMI Consumer Council: http://council.nami.org
National Association of State Mental Health Program Directors:
    www. nasmhpd.org
National Coalition of MH Professionals and Consumers:
    www.nomanagedcare.org
National Depressive and Manic-Depressive Association: www.ndmda.org
National Mental Health Association: www.nmha.org
President's New Freedom Commission: www.MentalHealthcommission.gov
Recovery, Inc.: www.recovery-inc.com
Substance Abuse & MH Services Administration (SAMHSA):
    http://mentalhealth.samhsa.gov
Treatment Advocacy Center: www.psychlaws.org
World Federation for Mental Health: www.icms.com.au/wfmh2003

# Appendix C
# Primary Archival Sources

Organizational Newsletters
  Consumer Supporter News (National Mental Health Association)
  Dendron News (Support Coalition International)
  The Key (National Mental Health Consumer Self-Help Clearinghouse)
  Labyrinth (M.C. Video Productions, Inc.)
  Madness Network News
  The Mental Health American (Mental Health America)
  MindFreedom Journal (Support Coalition International)
  National Empowerment Center Newsletter (Lawrence, Mass.)
  The Rights Tenet (National Association for Rights Protection and Advocacy)
  SafeTea (SAFE, Inc.)
  Second Opinion (Second Opinion Society)
  Vision (Pennsylvania Mental Health Consumers' Association)
  Multiple flyers and booklets received from movement individuals and organizations

Arts Publications and "Zines"
  Crazed Nation
  Transcendant Visions
  Reaching Across with the Arts (Altered States of the Arts)
  Multiple flyers and booklets received from movement individuals and organizations

Internet
  Numerous e-mail discussion groups, listservs, and websites (see Appendix B)

# Bibliography

*Adbusters: Journal of the Mental Environment. Mad Pride/Mad World Issue.* No. 41. Vancouver, BC, May/June 2002.

American Psychiatric Association. *Diagnostic and Statistical Manual of Mental Disorders,* 4th ed. Washington, DC: American Psychiatric Association, 1994.

Anspach, Renée. "From Stigma to Identity Politics: Political Activism among the Physically Disabled and Former Mental Patients." *Social Science & Medicine* 13A, (1979):765–773.

Barker, Phil, Peter Campbell and Ben Davison (eds.). *From the Ashes of Experience: Reflections on Madness, Survival and Growth.* London: Whurr Publishers, 1999.

Barry, Ellen. "Fisher named to mental health commission." *Boston Globe,* C2, 6/4/2002.

Bassman, Ronald. "Overcoming the Impossible: My Journey through Schizophrenia." *Psychology Today.* January/February (2001): 35–40.

Becker, Howard S. "Whose Side Are We On?" *Social Problems,* 14 (1967): 239–247.

Beers, Clifford Whittingham. *A Mind That Found Itself.* Pittsburgh: University of Pittsburgh Press, 1981.

Ben-Yehuda, Nachman. *Deviance and Moral Boundaries: Witchcraft, the Occult, Science Fiction, Deviant Sciences and Scientists.* Chicago: University of Chicago Press, 1985.

Borkman, Thomasina J. "Mutual Self-Help Groups: Strengthening the Selectively Unsupportive Personal and Community Networks of their Members. In *The Self-Help Revolution,* edited by F. Reissman and A. Gartner. New York: Human Sciences Press, 1984.

———. *Understanding Self-Help/Mutual Aid: Experiential Learning in the Commons.* New Brunswick, NJ: Rutgers University Press, 1999.

Breggin, Peter. *Toxic Psychiatry.* New York: St. Martin's Press, 1991.

———. *Brain-Disabling Treatments in Psychiatry: Drugs, Electroshock, and the Role of the FDA.* New York: Springer, 1997.

Breggin, Peter and David Cohen. *Your Drug May Be Your Problem: How and Why to Stop Taking Psychiatric Medications.* Reading, MA: Perseus Books, 1999.

Brown, Phil. "The Mental Patients' Rights Movement, and Mental Health Institutional Change." In *Mental Health Care and Social Policy,* edited by Phil Brown. Boston: Routledge, Kegan Paul, 1985.

Burstow, Bonnie and Don Weitz, (eds.). *Shrink Resistant: The Struggle Against Psychiatry in Canada.* Vancouver, BC: New Star Books, 1988.

Chamberlin, Judi. *On Our Own: Patient-Controlled Alternatives to the Mental Health System.* New York: Hawthorn Press, 1978

———. "The Ex-Patients' Movement: Where We've Been and Where We're Going." *Journal of Mind and Behavior* 11:3&4 (1990: 323[77]–336[90]).

Charlton, James I. *Nothing About Us Without Us: Disability Oppression and Empowerment.* Berkeley: University of California Press, 1998.

Charmaz, Kathy. *Good Days, Bad Days: The Self in Chronic Illness and Time.* New Brunswick, NJ: Rutgers University Press, 1991.

Chesler, Phyllis. *Women & Madness.* New York: Avon, 1972.

Church, Kathryn. *Forbidden Narratives: Critical Autobiography as Social Science.* Amsterdam: Gordon and Breach, 1995.

Curtis, Ted, Robert Dellar, Esther Leslie and Ben Watson (eds.). *Mad Pride: A Celebration of Mad Culture.* London: Spare Change Books, 2000.

Denzin, Norman. "Presidential Address on The Sociological Imagination Revisited." *The Sociological Quarterly,* 31(1990): 1–22.

Duerr, Maria. "Hearing Voices: Resistance among Psychiatric Survivors and Consumers." Masters Thesis. California Institute of Integral Studies, San Francisco, CA, 1996.

Emerick, Robert E. "Group Demographics in the Mental Patient Movement: Group Location, Age, and Size as Structural Factors." *Community Mental Health Journal* 25(1989): 277–300.

———. "Self-Help Groups for Former Patients: Relations with Mental Health Professionals." *Hospital and Community Psychiatry* 41(1990): 401–407.

———. "The Politics of Psychiatric Self-Help: Political Factions, Interactional Support, and Group Longevity in a Social Movement." *Social Science and Medicine,* 32(1991): 1121–1128.

———. "Clients as Claims Makers in the Self-Help Movement: Individual and Social Change Ideologies in Former Mental Patient Self-Help Newsletters." *Psychosocial Rehabilitation Journal* 18(1995): 19–35.

Erikson, Kai T. *Wayward Puritans: A Study in the Sociology of Deviance.* New York: John Wiley & Sons, 1966.

Estroff, Sue E. *Making It Crazy: An Ethnography of Psychiatric Clients in an American Community.* Berkeley: University of California Press, 1981.

Everett, Barbara. *A Fragile Revolution: Consumers and Psychiatric Survivors Confront the Power of the Mental Health System.* Waterloo, ON: Wilfrid Laurier University Press, 2000.

Farber, Seth. *Madness, Heresy and the Rumor of Angels: The Revolt against the Mental Health System.* Chicago: Open Court Press. 1993.

Favreau, Marie-Dianne Lucie. "The Pre-Shrinking of Psychiatry: Sociological InSights on the Psychiatric Consumer/Survivor Movement." Ph.D. Dissertation, University of California, San Diego, 1999.

Foucault, Michel. *Madness and Civilization: A History of Insanity in the Age of Reason.* New York: Random House, 1965.

———. *Power/Knowledge: Selected Interviews and other Writings 1972–1977,* edited by Colin Gordon. New York: Pantheon Books, 1970.

————. *The Birth of the Clinic: An Archaeology of Medical Perception.* New York: Random House, 1975.

————. *The History of Sexuality, Vol. 1: An Introduction.* New York: Random House, 1978.

————. *Discipline and Punish: The Birth of the Prison.* New York: Random House, 1979.

————. *Power,* edited by James D. Faubion. New York: The New Press, 1994.

Fox, Renée. *The Sociology of Medicine: A Participant Observer's View.* Englewood Cliffs, NJ: Prentice-Hall, 1989.

Frank, Leonard Roy (ed.). *The History of Shock Treatment.* San Francisco: Published by the author, 1978.

Freire, Paolo. *Pedagogy of the Oppressed.* New revised 20th anniversary edition. New York: Continuum, 1970/ 1994.

Freund, Paul. "Professional Role(s) in the Empowerment Process: 'Working With' Mental Health Consumers." *Psychosocial Rehabilitation Journal* 16:3(1993): 65–73.

Funk, Wendy. *What Difference Does it Make? (The Journey of a Soul Survivor).* Cranbrook, BC: Wildflower Publishing, 1998.

Gamson, William. *The Strategy of Social Protest.* 2nd Edition. Belmont, MA: Wadsworth Press, 1989.

Geertz, Clifford. *Local Knowledge: Further Essays in Interpretive Anthropology.* New York: Basic Books, 1983.

Geller, Jeffrey L. & Maxine Harris. *Women of the Asylum: Voices from Behind the Walls 1840–1945.* New York: Doubleday, 1994

Gerhardt, Uta. *Ideas about Illness: An Intellectual and Political History of Medical Sociology.* New York: New York University Press, 1989.

Goffman, Erving. *Stigma: Notes on the Management of Spoiled Identity.* New York: Simon & Schuster, 1963.

————. *Asylums: Essays on the Social Situation of Mental Patients and Other Inmates.* New York: Anchor Books, 1961.

Grob, Gerald. *The Mad among Us: A History of the Care of America's Mentally Ill.* Cambridge, MA: Harvard University Press, 1994.

Grobe, Jeanine (ed.). *Beyond Bedlam: Contemporary Women Psychiatric Survivors Speak Out.* Chicago, IL: Third Side Press, 1995.

Groch, Sharon. "Free Spaces: Creating Oppositional Consciousness in the Disability Rights Movement." In *Oppositional Consciousness: The Subjective Roots of Social Protest,* edited by Jane Mansbridge and Aldon Morris. Chicago: University of Chicago Press, 2001.

Hammersley, Martyn. *Taking Sides in Social Research: Essays on Partnership and Bias.* London: Routledge, 2000.

Haraway, Donna J. *Modest Witness @Second Millennium. FemaleMan Meets OncoMouse®: Feminism and Technoscience.* New York: Routledge, 1997.

Harp, Howie T. and Sally Zinman, (eds.). *Reaching Across II: Maintaining Our Roots/The Challenge of Growth.* Sacramento, CA: California Network of Mental Health Clients, 1994.

Hirsch, Sherry, et al. (eds.). *Madness Network News Reader.* San Francisco: Glide Publications, 1974.

hooks, bell. *Talking Back: Thinking Feminist, Thinking Black*. Boston, MA: South End Press, 1989.

Isaac, Rael Jean and Virginia C. Armat, *Madness in the Streets: How Psychiatry and the Law Abandoned the Mentally Ill*. New York: Free Press, 1990.

Johnstone, Lucy. *Users and Abusers of Psychiatry: A Critical Look at Psychiatric Practice*. 2nd ed. London: Routledge, 2000.

Kaufmann, Caroline L. "An Introduction to the Mental Health Consumer Movement." In *A Handbook for the Study of Mental Health: Social Context, Theories, and Systems*, edited by Allan V. Horwitz and Teresa L. Scheid. Cambridge: Cambridge University Press, 1999.

Klandermans, Bert. "The Social Construction of Protest and Multiorganizational Fields." In *Frontiers in Social Movement Theory*, edited by Aldon D. Morris and Carol McClurg Mueller. New Haven, CT: Yale University Press, 1992.

Kusow, Abdi. "Beyond Indigenous Authenticity: Reflections on the Insider/Outsider Debate in Immigration Research." *Symbolic Interaction* 26 (2003): 591–599.

Kusow, Abdi. "Contesting Stigma: On Goffman's Assumptions of Normative Orders." *Symbolic Interaction* 27 (2004): 179–197.

Lapon, Lenny. *Mass Murderers in White Coats: Psychiatric Genocide in Nazi Germany and the United States*. Springfield, MA: Psychiatric Genocide Research Institute, 1986.

Lemert, Edwin M. *Social Pathology*. New York: McGraw-Hill, 1951.

Levine, Bruce E. *Commonsense Rebellion: Debunking Psychiatry, Confronting Society*. New York: Continuum, 2001.

Lidz, Charles W., Alan Meisel and Mark Munetz. "Chronic Disease: The Sick Role and Informed Consent." *Culture, Medicine and Psychiatry* 9(1985): 241–255.

Lofland, John. *Deviance and Identity*. Englewood Cliffs, NJ: Prentice-Hall, 1969.

Lynch, Terry. *Beyond Prozac: Healing Mental Suffering without Drugs*. Dublin: Marino Books, 2001.

Mahler, Jay et al. "Letters: Taking Issue with Taking Issue: 'Psychiatric Survivors' Reconsidered." *Psychiatric Services* 48(1997): 601–605.

Maines, David R. "The Storied Nature of Health and Diabetic Self-Help Groups." *Advances in Medical Sociology*, Vol. 2(1991): 185–202.

Martensson, Lars. *Deprived of Our Humanity: The Case Against Neuroleptic Drugs*. Geneva, Switzerland: The Voiceless Movement, 1988.

McCubbin, Michael and David Cohen. "Extremely Unbalanced: Interest Divergence and Power Disparities between Clients and Psychiatry." *International Journal of Law & Psychiatry*, 19:1(1996): 1–25.

Melucci, Alberto. "Getting Involved: Identity and Mobilization in Social Movements." In *International Social Movement Research*, Vol. 1, edited by Bert Klandermans, Hanspeter Kriesi, and Sidney Tarrow. Greenwich, CT: JAI Press, 1989.

Millett, Kate. *The Loony-Bin Trip*. New York: Simon & Schuster, 1990.

Morrison, Linda. "Partial Success: In the Trenches of Mental Health Treatment." Unpublished paper, 1995.

———. "Communicating with Each Other: For a Change." Report on the Pittsburgh Dialogue on Mental Health Issues. Unpublished report, 1998.

———. "Committing Social Change for Psychiatric Patients: The Consumer/ Survivor Movement. *Humanity & Society* 24(2000): 389–404.

Mosher, Loren R. "Soteria: A Therapeutic Community for Psychotic Persons." In *Psychosocial Approaches to Deeply Disturbed Patients,* edited by P. Breggin and E.M. Sterns. New York: Haworth Press, 1996.

———. "Are Psychiatrists Betraying Their Patients?" *Psychology Today.* September/October, 40–41(1999): 80.

———. "Letter of Resignation from the American Psychiatric Association." Partially reprinted in *Adbusters: Journal of the Mental Environment.* 41, May/June 2002, no page number.

Naples, Nancy. "Deconstructing and Locating Survivor Discourse: Dynamics of Narrative, Empowerment, and Resistance for Survivors of Childhood Sexual Abuse." *Signs: Journal of Women in Culture and Society,* (28)2003: 1151–1185.

Nasar, Sylvia. *A Beautiful Mind.* New York: Simon & Schuster, 1998.

Newnes, Craig, Guy Holmes and Cailzie Dunn (eds.). *This is Madness: A Critical Look at Psychiatry and the Future of Mental Health Services.* Ross-on-Wye, UK: PCCS Books, 1999.

Omark, Richard. "The Dilemma of Membership in Recovery, Inc., a Self-help Mental Patients' Organization." *Psychological Reports,* 44:3(1979): 1119–1125.

Packard, Elizabeth. *The Prisoner's Hidden Life, or Insane Asylums Unveiled: As Demonstrated by the Report of the Investigating Committee of the Legislature of Illinois.* Chicago: Published by the Author, A.B. Case, 1868.

———. *Modern Persecution, or Married Woman's Liabilities.* Hartford, CT: Case, Lockwood & Brainard, 1874.

Parsons, Talcott. *The Social System.* Glencoe, IL: Free Press, 1951.

Porter, Roy. *A Social History of Madness: The World through the Eyes of the Insane.* New York: E.P. Dutton, 1987

Potok, Andrew. *A Matter of Dignity: Changing the Lives of the Disabled.* New York: Bantam Books, 2002.

Purinton, Linda (see also Morrison, Linda). "Mad Liberation: A Social Movement." Unpublished paper, 1993.

Reinarman, Craig. "The Twelve-Step Movement and Advanced Capitalist Culture: The Politics of Self-Control in Postmodernity." *In Cultural Politics and Social Movements,* edited by Marcy Darnovsky, Barbara Epstein and Richard Flacks. Philadelphia: Temple University Press, 1995.

Roth, Julius, *Timetables: Structuring the Passage of Time in Hospital Treatment and other Careers.* Indianapolis, IN: Bobbs-Merrill, 1963.

Satel, Sally L. *P.C., M.D.: How Political Correctness is Corrupting Medicine.* New York: Basic Books, 2000.

Sayce, Liz. *From Psychiatric Patient to Citizen: Overcoming Discrimination and Social Exclusion.* New York: St. Martin's Press, 2000.

Scheff, Thomas J. *Being Mentally Ill.* 2nd ed. Chicago: Aldine, 1966/1984.

———. *Being Mentally Ill: A Sociological Theory,* 3rd ed. New York: Aldine deGruyter, 1999.

Scholinksi, Daphne. *The Last Time I Wore a Dress: A Memoir.* New York: Riverhead Books, 1997.

Scott, James C. *Weapons of the Weak: Everyday Forms of Peasant Resistance.* New Haven, CT: Yale University Press, 1985.

———. *Domination and the Arts of Resistance: Hidden Transcripts.* New Haven, CT: Yale University Press, 1990.

Shimrat, Irit. *Call Me Crazy: Stories from the Mad Movement.* Vancouver, Canada: Press Gang Publishers, 1997.

Silverstein, Ken. "Prozac.org." *Mother Jones,* November/December (1999): 22–23.

Simmel, Georg. *On Individuality and Social Forms: Selected Writings,* edited by Donald N. Levine. Chicago, IL: University of Chicago Press, 1971.

Smith, Dorothy E. *The Everyday World as Problematic: A Feminist Sociology.* Boston, MA: Northeastern University Press, 1987.

Stefan, Susan. *Unequal Rights: Discrimination against People with Mental Disabilities and the Americans with Disabilities Act.* American Psychological Association, 2000.

Susko, Michael. *Cry of the Invisible.* Baltimore, MD: The Conservatory Press, 1991.

Szagedy-Maszak, Marianne. "Consuming Passion: The Mentally Ill are Taking Charge of Their Own Recovery. But They Disagree on What That Means," *U.S. News & World Report.* June 3, 2002: 55–57.

Szasz, Thomas. *The Manufacture of Madness.* New York: Dell Publishing, 1970.

———. *The Myth of Mental Illness: Foundations of a Theory of Conduct.* Revised edition. New York: Harper & Row, 1974.

———. *Law, Liberty and Psychiatry: An Inquiry into the Social Uses of Mental Health Practices.* Syracuse, NY: Syracuse University Press, 1989.

———. *Pharmacracy: Medicine and Politics in America.* Westport, CT: Praeger, 2001.

———. *Liberation by Oppression: A Comparative Study of Slavery and Psychiatry.* New Brunswick, NJ: Transaction Publishers, 2002.

Taylor, Verta. "Social Movement Continuity: The Women's Movement in Abeyance," *American Sociological Review* 54(1989): 761–75.

Torrey, E. Fuller. *Surviving Schizophrenia: A Family Manual* (revised edition). New York: Harper & Row, [1983] 1988.

———. *Out of the Shadows: Confronting America's Mental Illness Crisis.* New York: John Wiley & Sons, 1997a.

———. "Taking Issue: Psychiatric Survivors and Nonsurvivors," *Psychiatric Services* 48(1997b): 143.

———. "Hippie Healthcare Policy," *The Washington Monthly.* April 2002: 7–21.

Turner, Ralph. "The Theme of Contemporary Social Movements," *British Journal of Sociology* 20(1969): 390–405.

U.S. Department of Health and Human Services. *Mental Health: A Report of the Surgeon General-Executive Summary.* Rockville, MD: U.S. Department of Health and Human Services, Substance Abuse and Mental Health Services Administration. Center for Mental Health Services, National Institutes of Health, National Institute of Mental Health, 1999.

University of Pittsburgh Institutional Review Board. "Reference Manual for the Use of Human Subjects in Research. Pittsburgh, PA http://www.irb.pitt.edu/manual/default.htm

Unzicker, Rae. "On My Own: A Personal Journey through Madness and Re-Emergence," *Psychosocial Rehabilitation Journal,* 13(1989): 71–77.

Wechsler, Henry. "The Ex-patient Organization." *Journal of Social Issues,* 16:2(1960): 47–53.

Whitaker, Robert. *Mad in America: Bad Science, Bad Medicine, and the Enduring Mistreatment of the Mentally Ill.* Cambridge, MA: Perseus Publishing, 2002a.

———. "Mind Drugs may Hinder Recovery." *USA Today.* March 4, 2002, 13A, 2002b

Zinman, Sally, Howie the Harp, Su Budd (eds.). *Reaching Across: Mental Health Clients Helping Each Other.* Sacramento, CA: California Network of Mental Health Clients, 1987.

# Index

CPSIA information can be obtained
at www.ICGtesting.com
Printed in the USA
FSHW010626121219
64954FS

9 780415 804899